Paediatric Radiology for MRCPCH and FRCR

Christopher Schelvan
BSc MB BS MRCP FRCR
Specialist Registrar in Radiology,
The Middlesex Hospital,
UCL Hospitals, London

Annabel Copeman
BSc MB BS MRCPCH
Specialist Registrar in Paediatrics,
Great Ormond Street Hospital for Children, London

Jane Young
MSc MB BS FRCR
Consultant Radiologist,
The Whittington Hospital, London

Jacqueline Davis
MB BS FRCR
Consultant Radiologist,
The Whittington Hospital, London

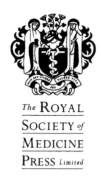

The ROYAL
SOCIETY of
MEDICINE
PRESS Limited

© 2002 Royal Society of Medicine Press Ltd

1 Wimpole Street, London W1G 0AE
207 Westminster Road, Lake IL 60045 USA
www.rsmpress.co.uk

British Library Cataloguing in Publication Data
A catalogue record for this book is available from the British Library

ISBN 1–85315–466–0

Typeset by Phoenix Photosetting, Chatham, Kent
Printed by Bell and Bain Ltd, Glasgow

Contents

Preface

Radiology plays an increasingly important role in the diagnosis and management of childhood diseases. This is reflected in both paediatric and radiology postgraduate exams, where candidates are expected to have a working knowledge of paediatric pathology, clinical manifestations, and appropriate radiological investigations.

The object of this book is twofold.

Our primary aim is to get you through your exams! With this in mind we have chosen examples of both important and common conditions, which a paediatrician and a radiologist should be able to recognize, and in which the imaging findings are typical and diagnostic. Though primarily concentrating on plain radiographs, we have used all the different imaging modalities to encompass many of the paediatric radiology cases that a candidate is likely to encounter. Some of the cases included are rare in clinical practice, but frequently turn up in exams.

The cases are randomly ordered to reflect the nature of the exams. Each case includes key points about the radiological and clinico-pathological aspects of the condition – the 'hot lists'. In this way we have tried to distil out the essence of each condition to complement the relative needs of a paediatrician and a radiologist in training.

The second objective is to give 'tools' in the form of methods for analysing some types of imaging modalities. These can be used when you don't have access to a paediatric radiologist.

This book does not aim to be a comprehensive guide to paediatric radiology – more of a whistle-stop-tour of classic films. We hope it helps you pass your exam.

Good luck!

Chris, Annabel, Jane and Jacky.

Foreword

For the inexperienced (and sometimes experienced) doctor, dealings with children, radiological interpretation and the appropriate use of a wide range of imaging modalities are areas prone to pitfalls.

The interpretation of children's X rays can be a daunting affair for both trainee paediatricians and radiologists, and the competences needed are acquired by reporting hundreds of routine and, not so routine films. This book distils many radiological pearls of wisdom, wraps them in a familiar clinical scenario, and enables the trainee to absorb the important facts and first principles by which radiological diagnoses are made.

This book is orientated towards candidates for MRCPCH and FRCR. It aims to provide the trainee with diagnostic clues with which to improve their interpretation of paediatric imaging – but not just for the purpose of passing examinations. More importantly, it provides a framework to make a radiological diagnosis, or assist in a difficult diagnosis when presented with similar scenarios in the middle of the night.

Not so much a reference book, more a 'radiologist in your pocket guide' to paediatric radiology, equipping you for the rigours of examinations, and improving the care of patients. I would recommend that all trainees (and a few consultants) keep a copy near to hand.

Andrew Raffles
MB BS FRCPCH FRCP DCH
Consultant Paediatrician and Regional Advisor in Paediatrics to the London Deanery
Queen Elizabeth II Hospital
E&N Herts NHS Trust
Welwyn Garden City, Herts

Acknowledgements

The authors would like to thank Dr Ranjana Chaudhury of the Whittington Hospital, London, and Dr Christine Hall of Great Ormond Street Hospital for Children, London, who provided some of the radiographs used in this book.

Rules and tools

1

How to look at a paediatric chest X-ray

HOW TO LOOK AT A PAEDIATRIC CHEST X-RAY

There is a lot of information on a chest X-ray and it helps to have a routine. This takes less time than you think and avoids basic mistakes, for example assessing the wrong patient. You will also start to look at all the information present instead of just looking at the heart and lung fields.

1. **Elementary stuff.** Check the name, date, side markers, and anything written on the film (e.g. 'film in expiration', 'lateral decubitus').
2. **Technical matters.** Ask yourself if the film is technically adequate. This sounds boring and unnecessary but this is why you must.

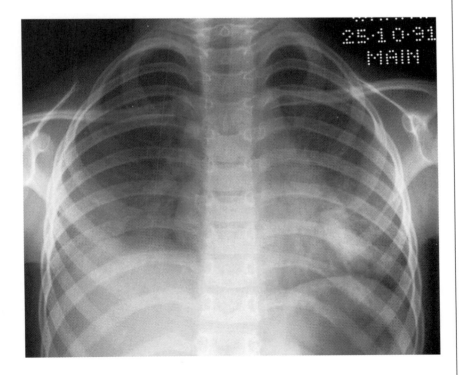

This child was admitted with a cough, and a chest X-ray was performed. What does it show? What is the diagnosis?

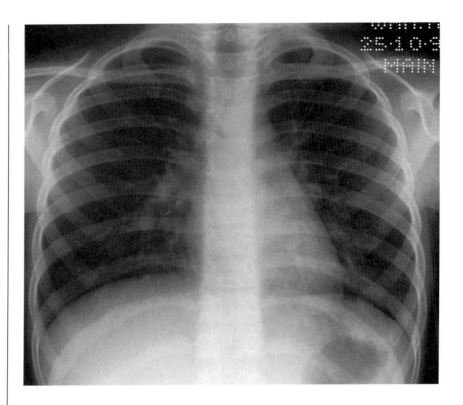

There is nothing the matter with the child's chest. The first film was taken in expiration (looking for air trapping). This film was taken immediately after the first one, and is in full inspiration. The lung fields are clear.

So you must assess the film for:

1. **Adequate inspiration**—five anterior ribs above the diaphragm.
2. **Rotation**—the medial ends of the clavicles should be equidistant from the spine.
3. **Penetration**—you should be able to see the spine through the heart.
4. Watch out for the **lordotic** projection—usually due to the child arching away from the cassette. This can result in distortion of the superior mediastinum, and apparent upper lobe blood diversion along with a boot-shaped heart.

Now you can interpret the film

Make sure you include all of these in your review (you may find it helps if you leave the heart and lungs until last).

(1) Bones: including spine, ribs and proximal humeri

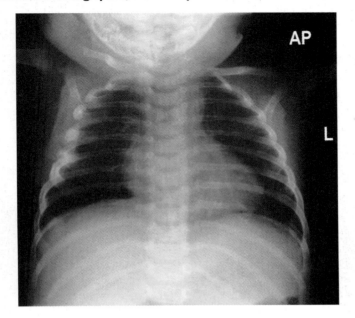

This child has a heart murmur: note the multiple vertebral abnormalities.

(2) Soft tissues

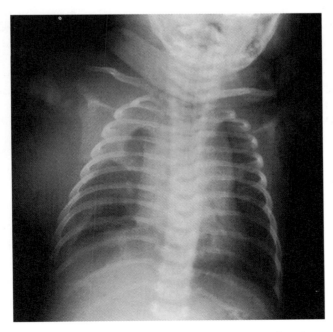

Note the soft tissue swelling over the right chest wall. This is due to a large haemangioma.

(3) Mediastinum including thymus

The thymus often causes difficulties in interpretation of the chest X-ray because of its variable size and configuration. Typically it lies on both sides of the superior mediastinum and has a smooth lateral border. It blends inferiorly with the cardiac contour, although sometimes there is a little notch at the junction. It is of low density, and lung markings can usually be seen through it. The normal thymus does not displace the trachea or oesophagus. On the plain film it is usually apparent until the age of 2, although it may be seen in older children (up to 4 years, and sometimes even older). The thymus may decrease in size in response to stress (e.g. infection) and return to normal when the child's clinical condition improves.

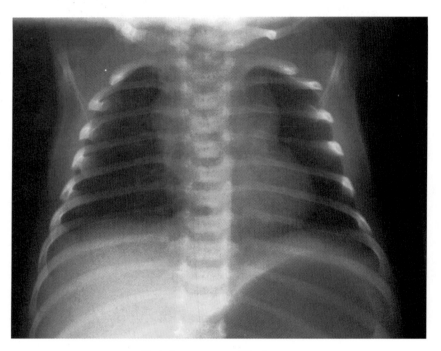

Typical appearances of the thymus.

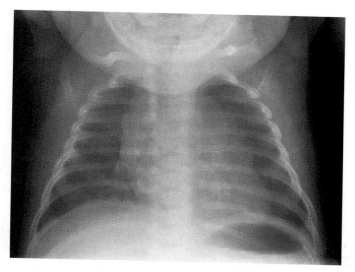

Typical appearances of the thymus.

(4) Heart

Assess the heart size but remember the film is usually taken AP. In infants the thymic outline may give a false impression of cardiomegaly. Note the position of the aortic arch and assess the pulmonary vasculature (plethora/oligaemia).

(5) Lungs

- Check the lung volumes:
  —Overinflated? (e.g. bronchiolitis).
  —Asymmetrical? (e.g. inhaled foreign body).
- Focal pathology—mass, collapse, consolidation.
- Diffuse abnormality—fibrosis, oedema.

Review areas (where you are likely to miss things) should include:

1. The superior mediastinum. A difficult area, especially in younger children because of the presence of the thymus. Make sure you don't mistake the thymus for lymphadenopathy/consolidation (and vice versa).
2. The hila—check their position (are they displaced by lobar collapse?) and their size and density.
3. Behind the heart—look for left lower lobe collapse/consolidation and paravertebral pathology.
4. Below the diaphragm—remember children may have a lot of air in their stomach, particularly if they have been crying, or have just had a feed before the examination.

Note: The apices are an important review area in adults, but apical pathology is less common in children. An opacity projected over the apex is more likely to be a hair plait than a mass lesion.

Remember to check the position of tubes and lines

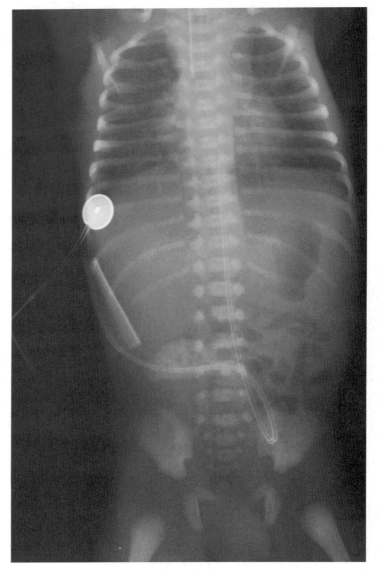

An umbilical artery catheter is present with its characteristic loop in the iliac artery in the pelvis. There is an endotracheal tube present.

Useful tips

1. Query any foreign body projected over the film—there is almost no small object that cannot be aspirated or swallowed.
2. Compare with previous films. Beware the child with a fat X-ray packet—they may have an underlying problem (e.g cystic fibrosis), which has been overlooked.

Nuclear medicine

These are the scans that look like huge numbers of dots coalesced to form a blurred shape. It is however an excellent functional imaging modality, used to assess the genitourinary, gastrointestinal, endocrine and musculoskeletal systems, and is of vital importance in paediatric radiology.

Renal nuclear medicine

This is the commonest type of paediatric nuclear medicine study performed in the district general hospital setting.

There are two types of renal scans:

1. **Static.** The tracer (DMSA) is taken up and retained by the kidney.
2. **Dynamic.** The tracer (MAG3 or DTPA) is taken up and excreted rapidly by the kidneys. Images of the renal tract are produced, and the passage of the tracer through the kidney is mapped by a graph, called a **renogram**.

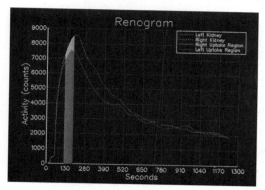

A normal renogram. The initial rise of the graph is the tracer arriving at the kidney through the bloodstream. The tracer then passes through the kidney, leading to the excretion (downward) part of the curve, when the tracer leaves the kidney in the urine.

In **obstruction**, the tracer accumulates in the collecting system and is not washed out.

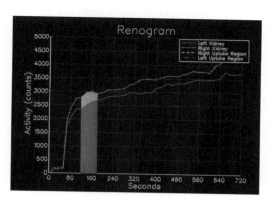

An obstructed renogram. The tracer arrives in the bloodstream (initial upward part of the graph). The graph continues to rise as tracer continues to arrive, but cannot leave the kidney.

Diuretics are necessary to confirm that this appearance is due to obstruction, rather than a 'baggy' slow-draining collecting system.

Nuclear cystogram

Used in the detection of vesicoureteric reflux. The cystogram can be direct, when the tracer is introduced directly into the bladder, or indirect, performed at the end of the standard renogram (voiding phase). A nuclear cystogram is preferred (where possible) to an X-ray cystogram as the radiation dose to the child is much less.

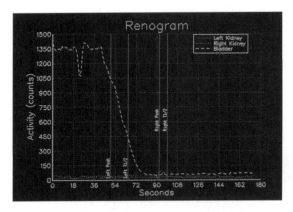

A normal cystogram. There is decreasing bladder activity during micturition, with no concurrent change in kidney activity.

An increase in the kidney activity during the voiding indicates reflux. Sometimes this is evident even prior to voiding. A small 'blip' at the end of voiding is often seen when reflux is present as tracer returns to the bladder from the kidneys.

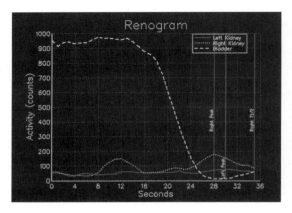

A cystogram showing vesicoureteric reflux. There is a concurrent rise in kidney activity during micturition as the bladder activity decreases.

STATIC SCANS

DMSA

This tracer is taken up by the renal parenchyma (proximal tubules). The study assesses functional renal tissue and is useful in:

- Assessment of scarring secondary to a urinary tract infection (UTI). Defects are better demonstrated than on a renogram.
- Detection of an abnormally located kidney.
- Assessment of renal function in abnormal kidneys, for example multi-cystic dysplastic kidney and pelvi-ureteric junction (PUJ) obstruction.

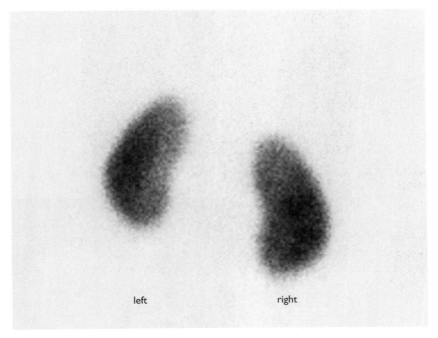

A normal DMSA scan. Note the reversed position of the kidneys due to posterior acquisition of the image.

Contrast studies

GASTROINTESTINAL STUDIES

Barium meal

- Usually performed looking for abnormalities of the oesophagus (e.g. reflux, vascular ring), and to exclude malrotation.
- Videofluoroscopy can be helpful in the investigation of children with feeding difficulties (e.g. assessment of swallowing and recurrent aspiration).

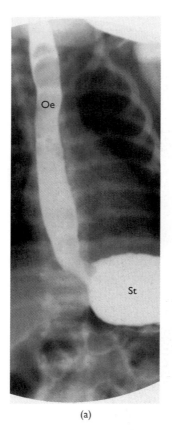

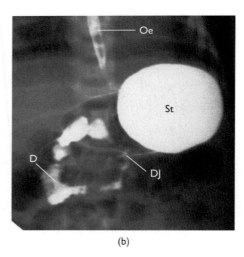

(a)   (b)

(a,b) Normal barium meal showing oesophagus, stomach, and duodenum. Oe = Oesophagus, St = Stomach, D = Duodenum, DJ = DJ Flexure.

Large bowel studies (barium or water-soluble contrast)

- Can be therapeutic (e.g. meconium ileus) or diagnostic (e.g. atresias, microcolon), or both (intussusception).

INTRAVENOUS UROGRAMS (IVU)

These are rarely performed, having been superceded by ultrasound. However they can occasionally be useful in defining anatomy, particularly in children with duplex systems.

MICTURATING CYSTOGRAM

Performed to look for reflux and to assess the urethra in boys. Whether these are done under direct screening or as nuclear medicine studies will depend on local practice.

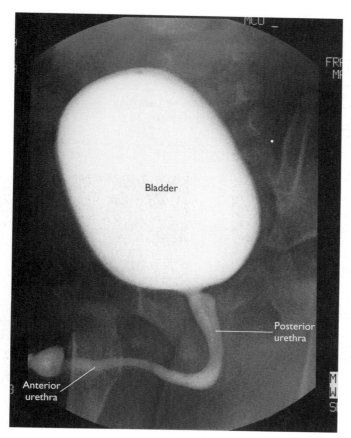

Normal cystogram in a boy.

Computed tomography (CT)

CT scans are those exciting radiology investigations that produce plenty of pictures and may require a radiologist to get out of bed in the night (request them with caution!).

PHYSICS FOR DUMMIES

CT is essentially a glamorous X-ray machine where both the X-ray beam and the detectors rotate around the patient in a spiral. X-rays shoot through the patient as the table moves continuously. The computer then generates an image from each rotation (**a slice**). Each slice contains data that can be manipulated to look at bone, soft tissue, lungs, and brain (**different windows**).

Basic concepts

Appearance of lesion on CT (soft tissue windows)	CT number (density or attenuation)	Causes
White	High	Bone, calcification, acute haemorrhage, contrast agents (intravenous or oral)
Intermediate grey	Intermediate (between +100 and −20)	Water, soft tissue
Black	Low	Fat, air

BUT REMEMBER:
The relative density of structures on CT depends on the window settings—the same structures will have completely different brightness levels on bone, lung and soft tissue windows.

ANATOMY FOR DUMMIES

We cannot teach you cross–sectional anatomy, but exams are all about 'classical pictures'—so learn to recognise normal anatomy on a few useful anatomical levels.

Chest

- Normal appearances are shown in the figures below.
- Recognise the normal mediastinal contours and the position of normal vascular structures (aorta and its main branches, superior vena cava, pulmonary arteries).

(a)
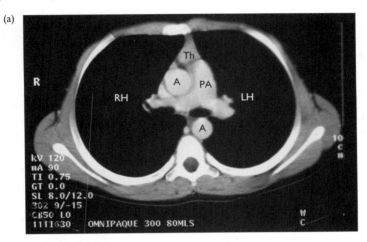

Contrast-enhanced CT chest at level of the hila. (a) Soft tissues windows. A = aorta, PA = pulmonary artery, RH = right hilum, LH = left hilum, Th = thymus.

(b)
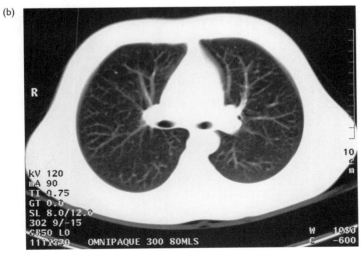

Contrast-enhanced CT chest at level of the hila. (b) Lung windows.

Abdomen
Normal appearances are shown below.

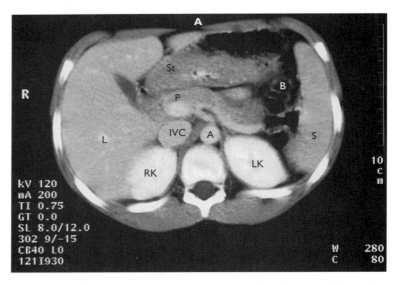

Contrast-enhanced CT of upper abdomen. L = liver, S = spleen, RK = right kidney, LK = left kidney, A = aorta, IVC = inferior vena cava, B = bowel, St = Stomach, P = Pancreas.

Brain
Normal CT appearances are shown below.

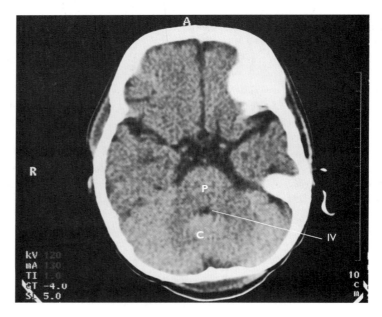

(a) Posterior fossa. C = cerebellum, P = pons, IV = IVth ventricle.

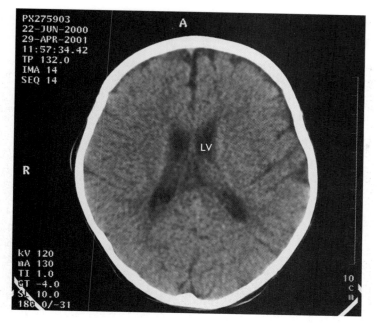

PX275903
22-JUN-2000
29-APR-2001
11:57:34.42
TP 132.0
IMA 14
SEQ 14

A

LV

R

kV 120
mA 130
TI 1.0
GT -4.0
SL 10.0
180 0/-31

10
C
m

(b) Cerebral hemispheres. LV = lateral ventricle.

Key points

- Be systematic—look at each organ in turn. Assess the size, and look for irregularities in contour and density of each organ. If you are looking at paired or symmetrical structures (kidneys, adrenals, brain) compare the two sides.
- Has contrast been given? Look at the blood vessels.
- In the absence of contrast, soft tissue high density represents calcification or haemorrhage.
- In the chest, look for abnormal soft tissue in the mediastinum (as a rule lymph nodes should not be greater than 1 cm in diameter) and lungs.
- In the abdomen look for abnormal soft tissue masses, free fluid and para-aortic lymphadenopathy (the 1 cm rule applies here too).
- In the brain, look for midline shift and make sure the lateral ventricles are a normal size and symmetrical. Low-attenuation lesions may represent tumours, infarcts, or oedema. Do not forget to have a quick look at the sinuses and orbits. Bone windows are important in trauma cases.

Magnetic resonance imaging (MRI)

MRI frightens everyone (including radiologists). It is a sophisticated non-radiation imaging modality that may eventually become the bread-and-butter of radiology.

PHYSICS FOR DUMMIES

MRI uses non-ionising magnetism instead of radiation. Different tissues contain different amounts of water (protons), so when a strong magnetic field is applied, the different tissues have different magnetic properties. This results in the exquisite soft tissue differentiation achieved with MRI.

T1 and T2 simply refer to different methods of sampling the magnetic resonance signal—meaning that the same soft tissue may have different signal characteristics on different sequences—for instance, fluid is low signal on T1 and high signal on T2.

The useful thing about MRI is that you can obtain images in any plane (the so-called 'multiplanar capacity' of MRI)—usually sagittal, coronal, or axial.

KEY POINTS

- MRI gives good soft tissue detail— useful in brain, spine and musculo-skeletal work. There is no signal from bone—use CT to evaluate bone pathology.
- **Fluid** (and therefore oedema surrounding masses or within inflamed areas) appears low signal (**dark**) on **T1** and high signal (**white**) on **T2**.
- **Gadolinium** (intravenous contrast) enhancement shows up as high signal areas (**white**) on T1 scans (if it enhances it's usually pathological).

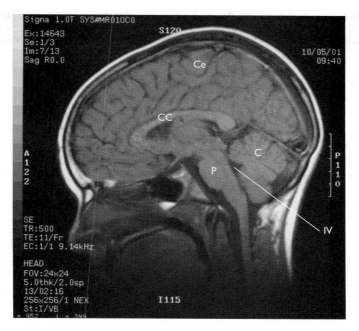

Sagittal T₁-weighted scan (note: CSF is dark). Ce = cerebral hemisphere, CC = corpus callosum, P = pons, C = cerebellum, IV = IVth ventricle.

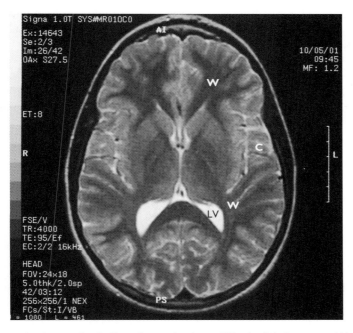

Axial T₂-weighted scan at level of lateral ventricles (note: CSF is bright). C = cortex, W = white matter, LV = lateral ventricle.

Selection of the appropriate imaging investigation

The battery of tests available increases year by year. Selection of a particular test depends on many factors. The availability, accuracy, degree of invasiveness and cost of the investigation will all influence the choice.

Remember some general principles:

1. The more information you give a radiologist, the better the quality of report you get. Discussing a sick/worrying child with the radiologist usually helps both parties. They are the experts in imaging, so use them.

2. The chance of a test yielding a positive result increases if the clinical evidence of the condition is high (known as a high pretest probability). For example, a child with abdominal pain is more likely to have appendicitis if they have a high white cell count, localised guarding and fever, than a child with vague abdominal pain and no fever. If the result of a test is surprising given the clinical findings, check your findings and discuss the case with the radiologist.

3. Some tests are very good at confirming or excluding the diagnosis, for example ultrasound for a hip effusion (a sensitive and specific test). Some tests are very good at telling you if something is present (sensitive) but a negative result does not exclude the diagnosis (not specific), for example CT scan for subarachnoid haemorrhage.

In general try to use non–invasive/non–radiation tests first.

Relative radiation dose of imaging investigations

Investigation	Radiation dose
Chest/abdomen X-ray	!
Skull X-ray	!!
Barium/contrast studies	!!!!!
Bone scan/Mag III	!!!!!
Ultrasound	None
CT head	!!!!!!!!!!!!
CT chest/abdomen	!!!!!!!!!!!!!!!!!!!!!!!!!!
MRI	None

Relative costs of imaging investigations

Investigation	Cost
Chest/abdomen X-ray	£
Cervical spine/skull	££
Barium/contrast studies	£££££££
Bone scan	£££££
Needle biopsy	£££££££££££
CT head	£££££££
CT chest/abdomen	£££££££
MRI	£££££££££££££££££££££££££

The cases

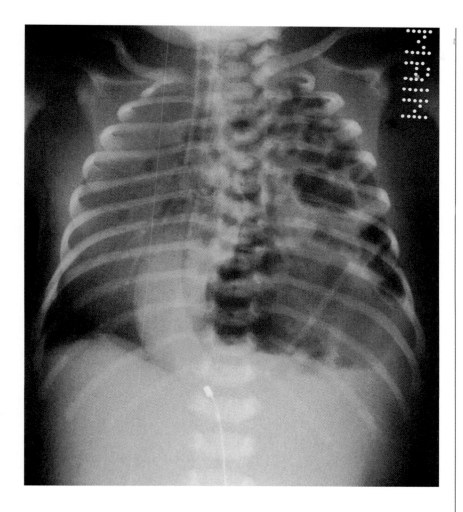

This term baby was admitted to the neonatal unit with respiratory distress.

1. What abnormalities are seen on the frontal chest radiograph?
2. What is the diagnosis?

ANSWERS

1. There are abnormal lucencies in the left hemithorax, representing bowel loops within the chest. There is mediastinal shift to the right and there is little aeration of the right lung. The gastric bubble is not seen in the normal position. The tip of the nasogastric tube is in the left chest.
2. Left congenital diaphragmatic hernia.

RADIOLOGY HOT LIST

- Initial radiographs may show a large and opaque hemithorax, as the bowel loops are fluid filled. As the baby swallows air, the characteristic gas-filled bowel loops appear in the thorax.
- Placement of a nasogastric tube verifies that there is bowel in the chest.
- The major differential diagnosis of cystic intrathoracic lesions is congenital cystic adenomatoid malformation, when there is a normal abdominal bowel gas pattern.

CLINICAL HOT LIST

- Incidence 1 : 4000 live births, most diagnosed antenatally.
- 80% of herniations are left posterolateral (Bochdalek).
- Embryology: the pleuroperitoneal opening (foramen of Bochdalek) fails to close. Abdominal viscera herniate into the thorax, compromising pulmonary development.
- Morbidity depends on the degree of pulmonary hypoplasia and associated pulmonary hypertension: the presence of aerated lung on both sides is a good prognostic indicator.

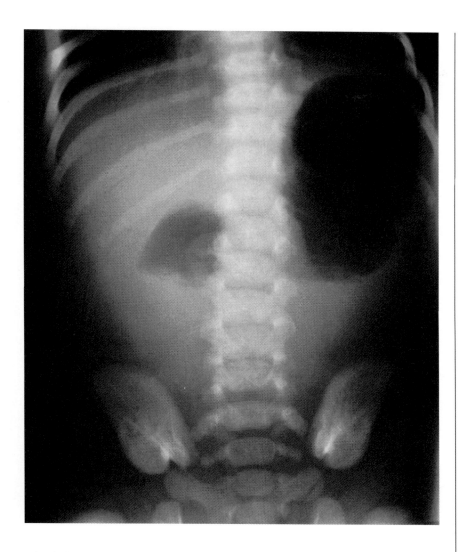

This baby was reviewed on the postnatal ward for poor feeding and bilious vomiting.

1. What abnormality is seen on the plain abdominal radiograph?
2. What is the most likely diagnosis?
3. With what condition is this associated?

ANSWERS

1. There is gas in the stomach and proximal duodenum but none else-where, giving the 'double bubble' sign.
2. Duodenal atresia.
3. Down's syndrome.

RADIOLOGY HOT LIST

- The abdominal X-ray is diagnostic and a contrast study is rarely required (danger of aspiration).
- The condition may be detected antenatally.
- If the abdominal radiograph suggests incomplete obstruction (with a small amount of gas in the distal bowel), a careful upper GI contrast study can be performed to assess the site of obstruction.
- Other causes of neonatal duodenal obstruction include duodenal stenosis, duodenal web, annular pancreas, Ladd's bands and midgut volvulus.

CLINICAL HOT LIST

- Incidence 1 : 3400 live births.
- Early developmental insult accounts for most cases. There is a high association with other abnormalities, e.g. anorectal, oesophageal, cardiac, and renal.
- Most atresias occur distal to the ampulla of Vater, thus causing bilious vomiting.
- Up to 30% have Down's syndrome.

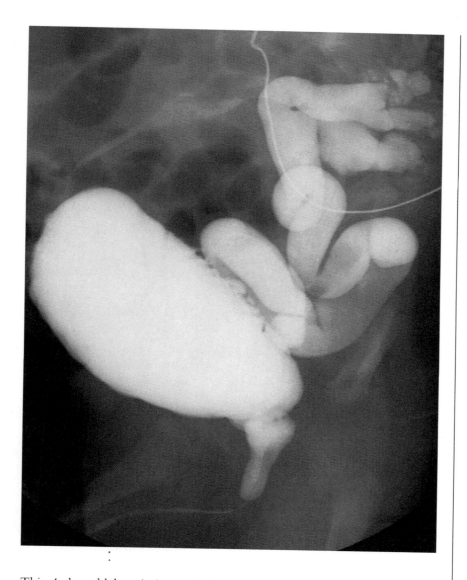

This 4 day old boy is in renal failure. Antenatal ultrasound had shown bilateral hydronephrosis.

1. What investigation is this?
2. What does it show?
3. What is the diagnosis?

ANSWERS

1. A micturating cysto-urethrogram (MCUG).
2. There is an abrupt change in calibre of the urethra, with dilatation of the posterior urethra. The bladder wall is trabeculated. There is bilateral vesicoureteric reflux into dilated and tortuous ureters. There is also intra-renal reflux.
3. Posterior urethral valves.

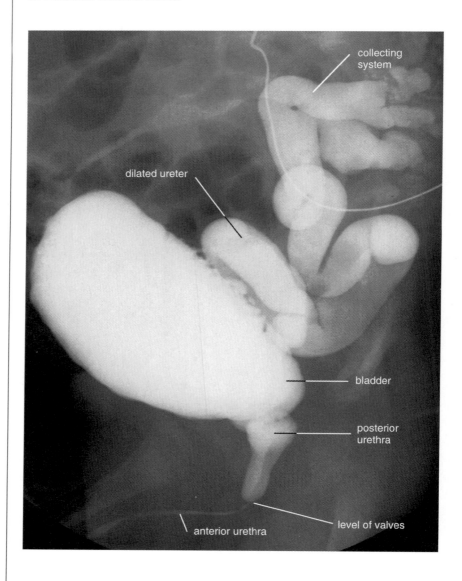

RADIOLOGY HOT LIST

- The diagnosis of posterior urethral valves is usually made on a MCUG. This will show dilatation of the posterior urethra, a transverse filling defect (valves), and reduction of the urethral calibre distal to the obstruction.
- There may be trabeculation of the bladder wall and a large residual volume.
- Vesicoureteric reflux is common, and is associated with a worse prognosis.
- Antenatal ultrasound may suggest the diagnosis, showing dilatation of the ureters and pelvicalyceal systems and a thick-walled, distended bladder. These findings in a male child should always prompt further assessment by MCUG.
- All children should be receiving prophylactic antibiotics at the time of the MCUG. The investigation should not be performed in the presence of a urinary tract infection.

CLINICAL HOT LIST

- Valves are mucosal folds, which close on voiding, leading to obstruction.
- It is the commonest obstructive uropathy in boys (1 : 8000). 40% present in the first 2 weeks of life, most before 6 months of age.
- Neonatal presentation may be with urinary retention, poor stream, infection or uraemia. Infants present more commonly with UTI.
- There is an association with renal dysplasia and 'prune belly' syndrome.
- Treatment is by surgical disruption of the valves. Prognosis depends on the duration and severity of obstruction prior to corrective surgery, and the presence of vesicoureteric reflux.

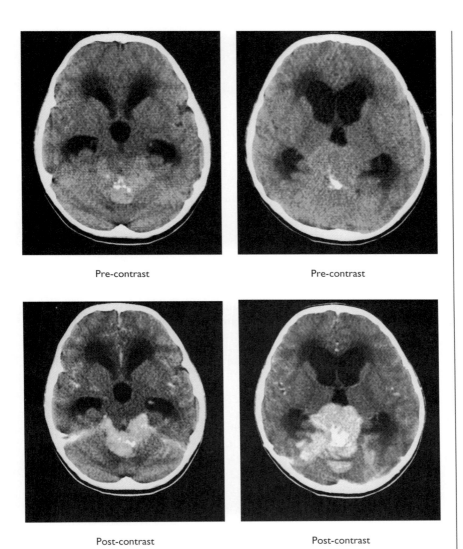

Pre-contrast

Pre-contrast

Post-contrast

Post-contrast

This 5 year-old boy was admitted with a 1 month history of headache and vomiting.

1. What does the CT scan show?
2. What is the most likely diagnosis?

ANSWERS

1. There is a midline solid mass in the posterior fossa, arising from the vermis and extending superiorly. It is partially calcified and shows marked enhancement after contrast. This is causing obstructive hydrocephalus (the periventricular low density indicates that this is acute).
2. Medulloblastoma.

RADIOLOGY HOT LIST

- Medulloblastoma is usually a well-defined posterior fossa mass arising from the cerebellar vermis in the midline. CT classically shows an intensely enhancing central solid mass.
- Encroachment on the IVth ventricle/aqueduct can cause hydrocephalus (present in 85–95%).
- Subarachnoid metastatic spread results in deposits in the spinal cord, cauda equina and intracranial CSF spaces. These are best assessed with MRI. Metastases also occur to bone, lymph nodes and lung.
- The differential diagnosis of childhood posterior fossa masses includes ependymoma, cerebellar astrocytoma, haemangioblastoma and brainstem glioma.

CLINICAL HOT LIST

- Medulloblastoma accounts for 20% of childhood CNS tumours (peak incidence 5 years).
- It commonly presents with signs of raised intracranial pressure secondary to obstructive hydrocephalus. Other features are progressive ataxia, diplopia, cranial nerve palsies, nuchal rigidity and head tilt.
- Prognostic features include tumour size, local extension and resectability, and presence of metastases.
- Treatment comprises surgical resection, and radiotherapy of the entire neural axis.
- 50% of patients will be disease free (with current treatment) at 5 years.

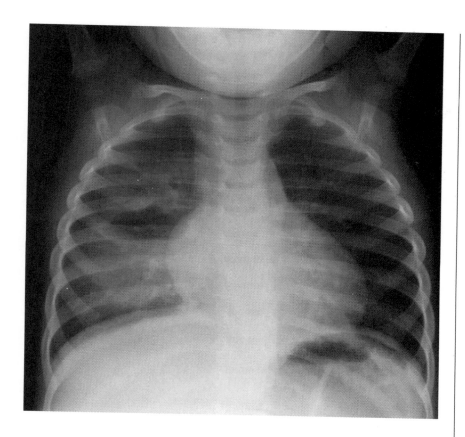

A 22 month old boy has a 2 week history of fever and cough, treated with antibiotics by his GP. On examination, he is miserable, febrile, with a tachycardia and tachypnoea.

1. What does the chest X-ray show?
2. What is the diagnosis?
3. What pathogens are most likely to be implicated?

ANSWERS

1. There is a cavity containing an air–fluid level in the right lower lobe (horizontal fissure visible, and right heart border preserved). There is surrounding consolidation.
2. A lung abscess.
3. Pathogens include *staphylococcus*, *klebsiella*, Gram–negative organisms and anaerobes (particularly if there is a history of aspiration).

RADIOLOGY HOT LIST

- Commonest sites: both upper lobes and the apical segments of the lower lobes, as these are dependent in recumbent patients.
- A CT scan may be necessary for exact localisation, and to distinguish an abscess from an empyema or a pneumatocele.
- Rupture of the abscess into the pleural space may cause an empyema or a pyopneumothorax.
- Lung abscesses may evolve into pneumatoceles (thin-walled cystic lesions) and persist for many months.

CLINICAL HOT LIST

- Lung abscesses are uncommon in children and are usually the sequelae of unresolved bacterial pneumonia, aspiration of foreign material, or disorders of host defence.
- Predisposing factors include: cystic fibrosis, endocarditis of the right heart, foreign body, immunodeficency and ciliary dyskinetic syndromes.
- Management is usually conservative, with intravenous antibiotics and radiological follow-up.
- Failure of resolution warrants bronchoscopy to identify obstructive lesions and to obtain bronchial aspirates for microbiological analysis.
- Drainage procedures are rarely required unless there is an empyema.

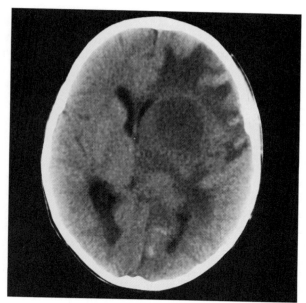

Pre-contrast

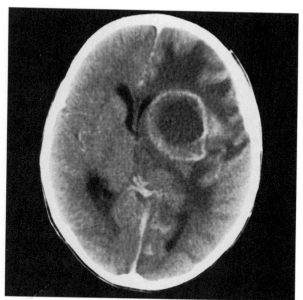

Post-contrast

This 8 year old boy was pyrexial and had a focal right-sided seizure. He had a 2 week history of sinusitis.

1. What abnormality is seen on the CT scan of the brain?
2. What is the diagnosis?

ANSWERS

1. There is a large ring-enhancing lesion surrounded by an area of low attenuation in the left frontal lobe. It is causing distortion of the anterior horn of the left lateral ventricle, and midline shift.
2. Left frontal cerebral abscess with surrounding cerebral oedema.

RADIOLOGY HOT LIST

- Non-contrast CT shows an area of low attenuation with mass effect, occasionally with increased rim density due to the abscess wall. Gas within the lesion is diagnostic of gas-forming organisms.
- Contrast-enhanced CT shows a ring-enhancing lesion with a smooth thick wall and surrounding oedema.
- MRI is the most sensitive modality for detecting further abscesses.

CLINICAL HOT LIST

- Causes of intracerebral abscess:
  —Suppuration in an adjacent anatomical structure, e.g. middle ear, sinuses.
  —Meningitis.
  —Distant source of infection, e.g. cyanotic congenital heart disease (R to L shunt), pulmonary suppuration.
  —Compound skull fracture or penetrating wound to cranium (including neurosurgery).
- Presentation is with headache, seizures, fever, altered level of consciousness. 70% have focal neurological signs.
- Cross-sectional imaging with contrast is the primary investigation. Lumbar puncture is dangerous and is not diagnostic.
- Management involves antibiotic therapy (including anaerobic cover) and neurosurgical consultation.

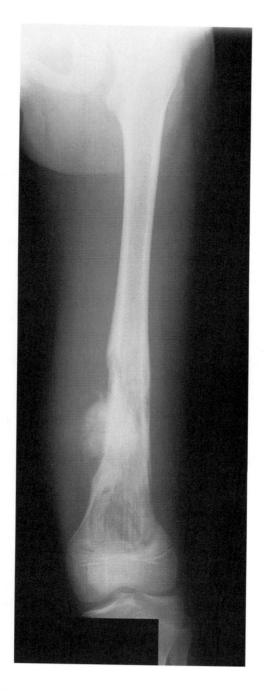

This 13 year old girl presented to A&E with a 1 month history of pain in the left knee.

1. What does the plain film show?
2. What is the most likely diagnosis?

ANSWERS

1. There is an ill-defined, destructive lesion in the distal femoral metaphysis. This is associated with extensive new bone formation and a lamellar periosteal reaction.
2. Osteosarcoma of the distal femur.

RADIOLOGY HOT LIST

- Osteosarcomas are most commonly located in the long bone metaphyses. Seventy per cent occur around the knee.
- They may be sclerotic or lytic lesions. They are aggressive in appearance with poorly defined margins, cortical disruption and with a wide zone of transition between normal and abnormal bone.
- There is a periosteal reaction which is ill-defined and irregular, often with an associated ossifying soft tissue mass.
- MRI is required to evaluate bone marrow extension, vascular involvement, and the soft tissue component.
- A bone scan will demonstrate bony metastases, while chest CT is required to exclude pulmonary metastases (the most common site).

CLINICAL HOT LIST

- Osteosarcoma accounts for 60% of malignant bone tumours in childhood, M > F, peak incidence second decade.
- It arises from primitive mesenchymal stroma.
- Predispositions and associations − chronic osteomyelitis, previous radiotherapy, retinoblastoma and chromosome 13 defect.
- Treatment: surgical excision and chemotherapy.
- Five year survival is 65% if there are no metastases at presentation.

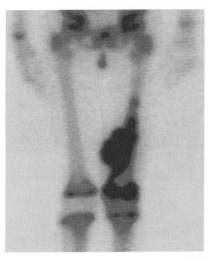

Bone scan shows the primary tumour in the distal left femur.

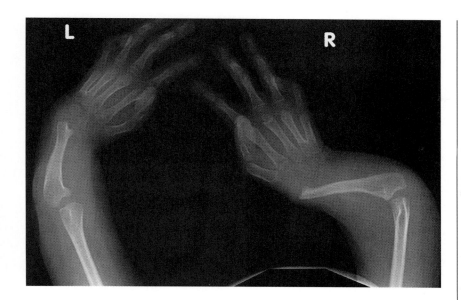

This child bruises easily.

1. What abnormality is seen on the X-ray of the forearms and hands?
2. What is the diagnosis?

ANSWERS

1. The radius is absent and the ulna is short on both sides. Both thumbs are hypoplastic.
2. Thrombocytopenia–Absent Radius (TAR) syndrome.

RADIOLOGY HOT LIST

- Aplasia/hypoplasia of the radius is one of several limb reduction anomalies. Radial ray anomalies refer to the radius, first metacarpal, and thumb.

CLINICAL HOT LIST

- Inheritance is mostly sporadic.
- Absent radius is associated with:
  —Thromboctyopenia–Absent Radius (TAR) syndrome.
  —Fanconi's anaemia.
  —Holt–Oram syndrome.
  —VATER/VACTERL.
  —Acrofacial dysostosis.

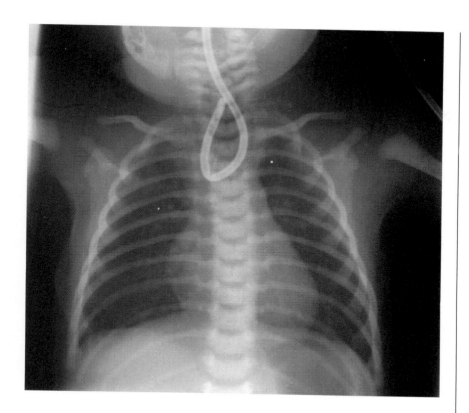

This 6 hour old baby was admitted to the neonatal unit with choking and cyanosis during his first feed.

1. What abnormality is seen on the chest radiograph?
2. What is the diagnosis?

ANSWERS

1. The nasogastric tube is coiled in a blind-ending proximal oesophageal pouch. The gastric air bubble is present. The lungs are clear, with no evidence of aspiration.
2. Oesophageal atresia with a tracheo-oesophageal fistula.

RADIOLOGY HOT LIST

- The site of the atresia is usually apparent, though air can be injected to distend the blind-ending pouch (usually at the junction of the upper one-third and lower two-thirds of the oesophagus).
- The presence of air in the stomach is indicative of a tracheo-oesophageal fistula.
- Avoid contrast studies when oesophageal atresia is present, as there is a significant risk of aspiration.
- An oesophagogram study is required to identify an H-type fistula (2%), when there is a normally patent oesophagus.
- Remember the VATER/VACTERL association and look for other anomalies.

CLINICAL HOT LIST

- Incidence is 1:3000, with associated malformations in up to 50%.
- There are five anatomical variants (85% have oesophageal atresia with a distal tracheo-oesophageal fistula).
- Nurse prone and head up, with a Repolge tube on suction in the oesophageal pouch to prevent aspiration.
- Surgical repair depends on oesophageal length: primary end-to-end anastomosis, or a staged repair to allow growth of segments, followed by gastric/colonic interposition.

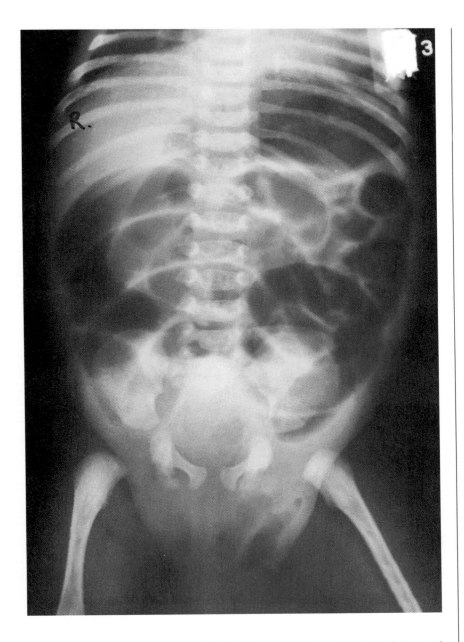

This 3 month old boy was seen in A&E with inconsolable crying, abdominal distension and vomiting.

1. What abnormalities are seen on the abdominal radiograph?
2. What is the diagnosis?

ANSWERS

1. There are centrally located and dilated bowel loops, with no gas in the rectum. There is a gas shadow projected over the scrotum. No free air seen.
2. Small bowel obstruction secondary to a left inguinal hernia.

RADIOLOGY HOT LIST

- It is difficult to distinguish between small and large bowel in young children. Clues include anatomical location (central loops more likely to be small bowel) and presence of complete mucosal folds (small bowel) or incomplete haustra (large bowel).
- If the distended bowel loops are fluid filled, the abdomen may have a 'gasless' appearance.
- Always look for intrascrotal air as incarcerated hernias are the most common cause of small bowel obstruction in infants under 6 months (excluding the neonatal period).
- Look for free intraperitoneal air secondary to perforation.

CLINICAL HOT LIST

- Adhesions are the most common cause of obstruction in babies who have had previous neonatal surgery.
- Other causes of obstruction to consider include extrinsic masses (e.g. tumour or appendix abscess), intussusception, Ladd's bands, and small bowel volvulus secondary to malrotation.

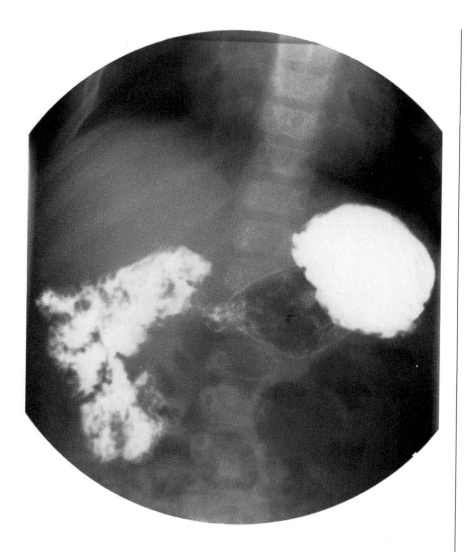

A 2 day old boy is reviewed on the postnatal ward. Breast-feeding is well established and he has passed a small amount of meconium on day one. There is now a 6 hour history of bile-stained vomiting.

1. What is this study?
2. What abnormality is demonstrated?
3. What is the diagnosis?

ANSWERS

1. An upper gastrointestinal contrast study.
2. The duodeno-jejunal (DJ) flexure and proximal small bowel loops are abnormally sited, lying to the right of the midline.
3. Malrotation.

RADIOLOGY HOT LIST

- An upper GI contrast study is the definitive investigation to identify the presence and location of an obstruction.
- The position of the duodeno-jejunal flexure is critical in the diagnosis of malrotation. It should lie to the left of the midline, at the level of the pylorus. The proximal jejunal loops should be left sided.

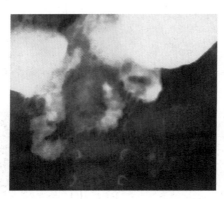

Upper GI contrast study showing normally sited DJ flexure.

- Mid-gut volvulus may occur, resulting in the small bowel having a 'corkscrew' appearance, as it twists around the superior mesenteric artery.
- Reversal of the position of the superior mesenteric artery and vein on ultrasound may suggest malrotation, but is not definitive.

CLINICAL HOT LIST

- Malrotation is a neonatal surgical emergency and needs to be excluded in neonatal bilious vomiting.
- Malrotation is an abnormality of small bowel rotation and fixation. The normal small bowel mesentery should be fixed from the DJ flexure in the left upper quadrant to the caecum in the right iliac fossa. In malrotation the mesentery is abnormally sited and narrow, allowing the small bowel to twist around a narrow pedicle (a volvulus).
- The superior mesenteric artery is contained in the twisted mesentery, leading to small bowel ischaemia and potential infarction.
- Obstruction may be intermittent, and the diagnosis should be considered in older children with similar symptoms.

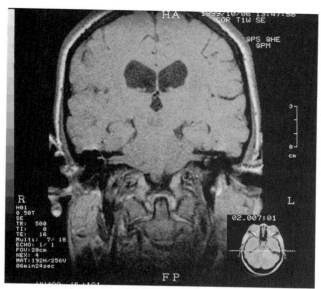

(a) Pre-contrast

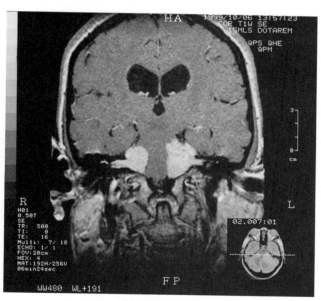

(b) Post-contrast

This 14 year old girl, with an inherited disorder, had a progressive onset of bilateral sensory neural deafness. An MRI brain scan was obtained.

1. What abnormalities are seen on the coronal T1–weighted images pre- and post-enhancement?
2. What is the diagnosis?
3. What is the underlying condition?

ANSWERS

1. There are bilateral isointense masses (on T1 weighting) at the cerebello-pontine angles, which show intense enhancement with gadolinium. The masses extend into and expand the internal auditory canals bilaterally. The pons is compressed.
2. Bilateral acoustic neuromas.
3. Neurofibromatosis type 2.

RADIOLOGY HOT LIST

- Acoustic neuromas are schwannomas, which arise from the vestibular (VIII) nerve. They may arise within, or at the opening of the internal auditory canal, and classically expand and erode the internal acoustic meatus.
- There may be obliteration of the ipsilateral cerebellopontine (CP) angle cistern, compression of the pons and distortion of the IVth ventricle with associated hydrocephalus.
- The mass is usually non-calcified, and shows intense enhancement on both CT and MRI.
- Acoustic neuromas account for 80% of CP angle tumours. Other causes include meningiomas and dermoid tumours.

CLINICAL HOT LIST

- Bilateral acoustic neuromas allow a presumptive diagnosis of neuro-fibromatosis type 2 (NF2).
- NF2 is an autosomal dominant disorder, distinct from NF1. Gene location: chromosome 22q.
- Clinical features of acoustic neuromas are slowly progressive deafness, imbalance, tinnitus, cerebellar ataxia, features of raised intracranial pressure and other cranial nerve palsies.
- NF2 is associated with a few café–au–lait spots (<5), and subcutaneous neurofibromas (minimal in size and number). Meningiomas and ependy-momas also occur.

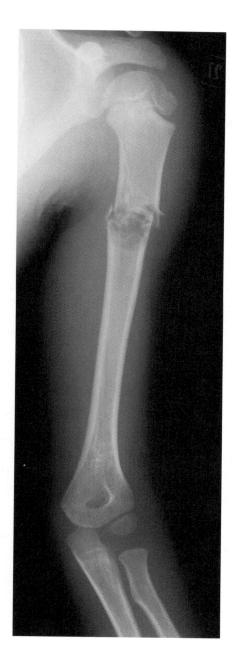

This 4 year old boy presented to A&E with pain in the left upper arm following a relatively trivial fall.

1. What does the X-ray show?
2. What is the most likely diagnosis?

ANSWERS

1. There is a fracture through the proximal humerus at the site of a well-defined lytic lesion.
2. A pathological fracture through a simple bone cyst.

RADIOLOGY HOT LIST

- Simple bone cysts are characteristically well-defined, expanded lytic lesions, with a thin but intact bony cortex.
- They are commonly found in the proximal humerus and proximal femur, and are usually asymptomatic unless a pathological fracture occurs. They may be incidental findings on plain radiographs.
- Fibrous dysplasia can mimic these appearances radiologically.

CLINICAL HOT LIST

- Simple bone cysts originate at the epiphyseal plate in long bones and grow into the shaft of the bone, changing position with skeletal maturity. They are rarely seen after the age of 30.
- If symptomatic they may require curettage and bone packing.

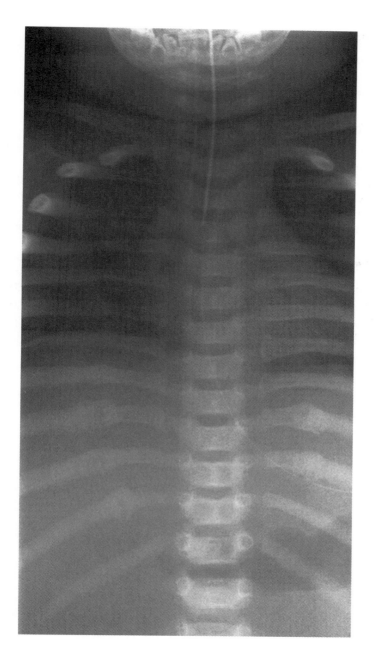

This baby was admitted having collapsed at home. There was a history of a visit to another casualty department with a similar episode. This is a post-intubation film.

1. What abnormality is seen on the chest X-ray?
2. What is the significance?
3. What further imaging should be performed?

ANSWERS

1. There are healing fractures of the posterior ribs on both sides.
2. This is highly suggestive of non-accidental injury (NAI).
3. A dedicated skeletal survey will be required.

RADIOLOGY HOT LIST

- Rib fractures in children under the age of 2 years are almost always due to NAI.
- Rib fractures are rare in childhood as the compressive forces required are considerable. Unless there is a history of significant trauma (e.g. road traffic accident) always be suspicious.
- Posterior rib fractures are specific for NAI. They result from severe compression of the rib cage, usually during a shaking episode.
- Rib fractures may not be visible immediately, but delayed films at 10 days will show callus formation and periosteal reaction. Always consider delayed films if there is a high index of suspicion with a normal chest X-ray. A bone scan may be positive within hours of injury and may reveal other injuries.

CLINICAL HOT LIST

- The reported incidence of NAI varies, from 15 to 42 cases per 1000 children. It is likely that there is significant underreporting of child abuse.
- It is a major cause of morbidity and mortality.
- Young children may present with collapse or near-miss cot death due to cerebral injury.
- There is often inadequate explanation for injuries, inconsistencies in the history and delayed presentation.
- There may be multiple injuries with presentation to different hospitals.
- After dealing with the injuries, management is to keep the child in a place of safety with assessment by the child protection team.
- Outcome: death 2%, severe injury 30%, re-injury 10–30%, returned to family 60%.

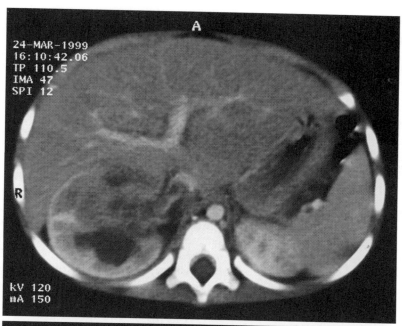

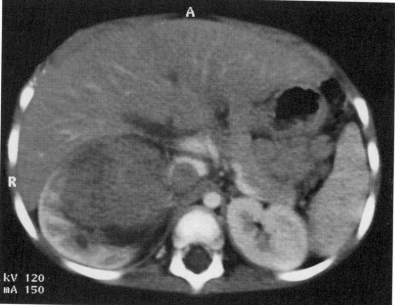

The parents of this 3 year old boy noticed an abdominal mass when they were giving him a bath.

1. What abnormalities are seen on this contrast-enhanced CT scan of the abdomen?
2. What is the diagnosis?
3. What are the associated risk factors for this condition?

ANSWERS

1. There is a large, non-enhancing and mixed-attenuation mass arising from the right kidney. No calcification is seen. There is a filling defect within the right renal vein and inferior vena cava (IVC) representing tumour invasion. The other blood vessels are displaced by the mass. The liver and left kidney appear normal on these images.
2. Wilms' tumour.
3. Chromosome 11 point deletion, aniridia, hemihypertrophy, genitourinary abnormalities, Beckwith–Wiedemann syndrome, Drash syndrome.

RADIOLOGY HOT LIST

- Wilms' tumours are bilateral in 5%.
- The tumour usually has well-defined margins and classically **displaces** adjacent vessels, as opposed to encasing them (as with neuroblastoma).
- 5% have tumour thrombus in the renal vein and IVC.
- The plain abdominal radiograph may show enlargement of the renal out-line and displacement of the adjacent bowel gas. Calcification is rare (10%).
- Chest CT is used to detect pulmonary metastases (present in 10% at diagnosis).

CLINICAL HOT LIST

- Incidence 1 : 10 000 live births, M = F, most under 7 years (peak 3 years).
- Presentation is usually in a well child with a non-tender abdominal mass. 25% have haematuria, 5% hypertension.
- Staging of disease:

Stage		10 year survival
I	One kidney, capsule intact, complete excision	95%
II	Extension beyond capsule, complete excision	87%
III	Residual tumour within abdomen	81%
IV	Haematogenous spread, e.g. lung, bone, liver	62%
V	Bilateral renal tumours	73%

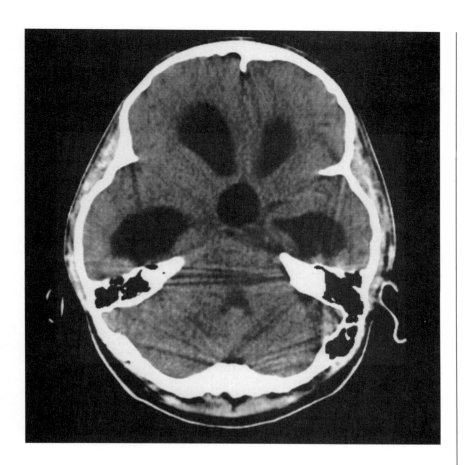

This 8 year old boy has a large head and mild developmental delay.

1. Describe the abnormalities on the CT scan.
2. What is the condition?
3. What is the most likely cause?

ANSWERS

1. There is marked dilatation of the lateral and third ventricles with a normal size fourth ventricle. There is no mass lesion.
2. Non-communicating hydrocephalus.
3. Congenital aqueduct stenosis.

RADIOLOGY HOT LIST

- Dilatation of the lateral (note the dilated temporal horns) and third ventricles with a normal size fourth ventricle indicates that the level of obstruction is at the aqueduct of Sylvius.
- Congenital aqueduct stenosis is the commonest cause of congenital hydrocephalus.
- There is no periventricular low density (which would indicate acute hydrocephalus), implying a longstanding abnormality.

CLINICAL HOT LIST

- Hydrocephalus is due to an imbalance of CSF production and reabsorption.
- Obstructive hydrocephalus is due to obstruction of the normal CSF flow and/or reabsorption. Overproduction of CSF (secondary to choroid plexus papilloma) is rare.

Type of obstructive hydrocephalus	Pathophysiology	Example
Communicating	Extraventricular blockage occurs beyond the fourth ventricle within the subarachoid pathways and arachnoid granulations. All ventricles dilated	Post-meningitis, post-haemorrhage
Non-communicating	Ventricular blockage with dilatation of ventricles proximal to obstruction.	Arnold–Chiari II malformation, Dandy–Walker malformation, vein of Galen aneurysm, tumour

- The clinical presentation will vary with age and aetiology. Chronic presentation may include increasing head circumference, developmental delay and behavioural changes. An acute decompensation may present with signs of raised intracranial pressure, seizures and acute squint.
- Management involves neurosurgery and ventricular shunting.

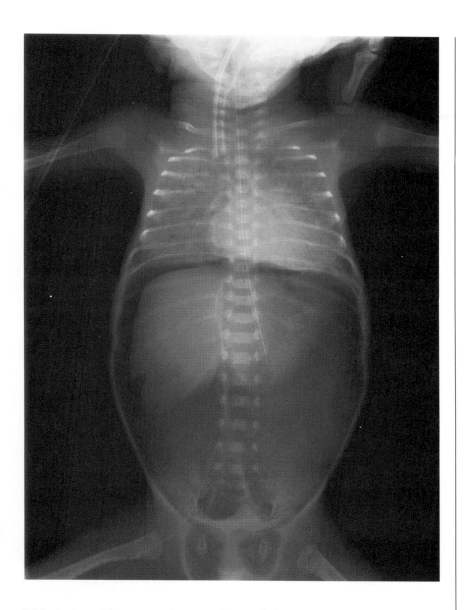

This 5 day old neonate, born at 27 weeks' gestation and ventilated for hyaline membrane disease, has abdominal distension, metabolic acidosis and cardiovascular collapse.

1. What does the abdominal radiograph show?
2. What is the diagnosis?

ANSWERS

1. There is a large amount of free intraperitoneal air present, which outlines the diaphragm and liver. There is air in the scrotum (bilateral patent processus vaginalis). The bowel loops are not well seen. There is an endotracheal tube, NG tube and umbilical vein catheter in situ. Both lungs show patchy infiltrates.
2. Acute GI perforation (usually secondary to necrotising enterocolitis). This baby survived.

RADIOLOGY HOT LIST

- Free intraperitoneal air may not lie under the diaphragm when the patient is supine. Free air will collect in the least dependent area (adjacent to the anterior abdominal wall), resulting in a central rounded lucency ('football sign'). This may be quite subtle.

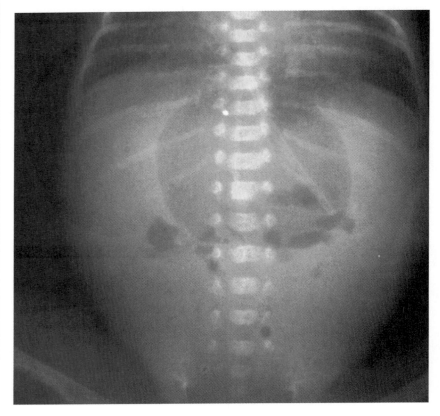

GI perforation showing football sign.

- Air may outline the falciform ligament which appears as a dense linear opacity (due to free air either side of it) in the midline or right upper quadrant.
- The bowel wall may be seen clearly as a thin white line if there is air on both sides of it (Rigler's sign). Look for intrascrotal air in premature babies.
- A horizontal beam 'shoot-through' film of the supine baby will show free air adjacent to the anterior abdominal wall in equivocal cases.

CLINICAL HOT LIST

- Major causes of neonatal perforation include necrotising enterocolitis, Hirschsprung's disease, bowel atresia, imperforate anus and meconium ileus.

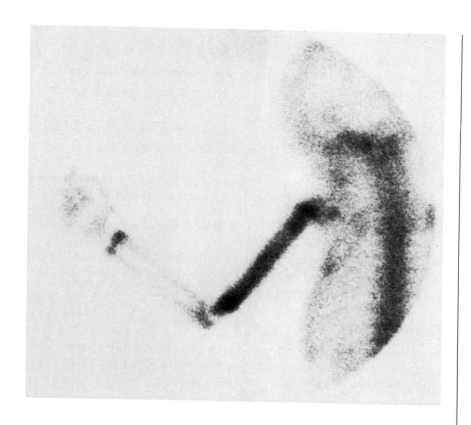

A 4 year old Afro-Caribbean girl was brought to the A&E department with a high temperature and a painful right arm. The arm was tender and erythematous. The X-ray is normal.

1. What is this investigation?
2. What does it show?
3. What is the diagnosis?

ANSWERS

1. Bone scan using technetium-99m MDP.
2. There is increased uptake of tracer throughout the right humerus.
3. Osteomyelitis.

RADIOLOGY HOT LIST

- X-rays are usually normal in acute osteomyelitis, and it may take up to 10 days before plain film changes are seen.
- A bone scan is usually the first-line investigation, and is generally positive within hours of the clinical signs appearing. It is useful to identify the site(s) of the infection.
- A white cell scan can be used to confirm pyogenic osteomyelitis where the bone scan is equivocal.
- MRI will demonstrate the soft tissue extent of the infection. It is as sensitive for osteomyelitis as the bone scan, but cannot cover the entire skeleton, and may require sedation.

CLINICAL HOT LIST

- Osteomyelitis occurs secondary to haematogenous spread or penetrating injury. Chronic presentation may be due to failed/ inadequate treatment or underlying immunodeficiency.

Population	Organism
Infant	*Staphylococcus aureus*, group B *Streptococcus*, Gram-negative bacteria
Child	*S. aureus* (70%), *Streptococcus*, *Haemophilus*
Sickle cell disease	*Salmonella*
TPN dependent	*Candida*

- It presents with sudden onset of local pain, swelling, erythema, and immobility. The child is systemically unwell with fever and malaise. Blood cultures are positive in 50%.
- Parenteral bacteriocidal antibiotics are needed initially. Six weeks of antibiotic therapy are usually required to eradicate infection. Early orthopaedic involvement is necessary as surgical decompression may be required, and may aid a microbiological diagnosis.

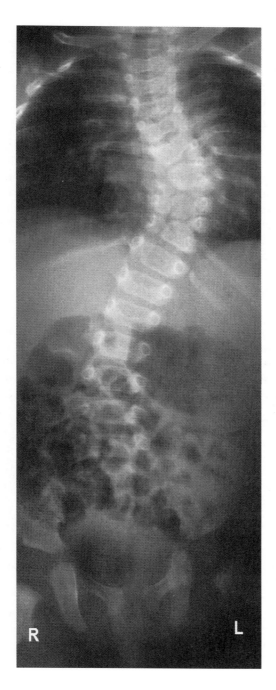

This baby was operated on in the neonatal period for anorectal atresia, and has absent radii. This radiograph of the spine was taken at 4 months of age.

1. What abnormality is seen on the plain radiograph?
2. What is the underlying diagnosis?

ANSWERS

1. There is a thoracolumbar scoliosis centred at T8/9, which is concave to the right. There are multiple abnormal vertebrae between T6 and T11.
2. VATER or VACTERL association.

RADIOLOGY HOT LIST

- Scoliosis is a lateral curvature of the spine, which may be structural (loss of lateral bending ability) or non-structural (normal mobility).
- Causes include: idiopathic (most common), congenital, neuromuscular disease, skeletal dysplasias, post-traumatic, post-inflammatory.
- Congenital scoliosis is due to vertebral abnormalities, with a progressive curve and often requiring operative intervention.
- Congenital scoliosis is often associated with other anomalies, particularly cardiac and genitourinary.

CLINICAL HOT LIST

- VATER and VACTERL are associations; combinations of congenital abnormalities that occur at a higher frequency than by chance alone.
- **V**ertebral anomalies, **A**nal atresia, **T**racheo**E**sophageal, **R**adial, **R**enal abnormalities.
- **V**ertebral, **A**norectal, **C**ardiac, **T**racheo**E**sophageal, **R**enal and **L**imb abnormalities.

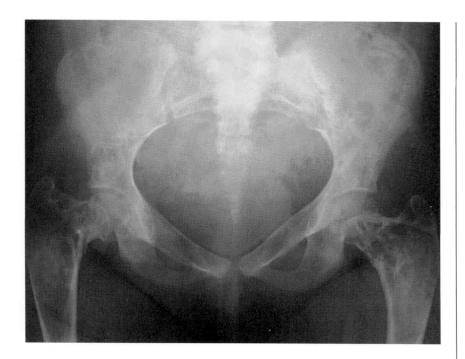

This 9 year old girl has right hip pain, hyperpigmented areas of skin, and precocious puberty.

1. What does the plain X-ray of the pelvis show?
2. What is the diagnosis?
3. What is the underlying condition?

ANSWERS

1. There are well-defined, expansile lytic lesions in both proximal femora resulting in bilateral coxa vara. Similar lesions are seen in the iliac bones. There is no breach in the cortex, periosteal reaction, or associated soft tissue mass.
2. Polyostotic fibrous dysplasia.
3. McCune–Albright syndrome.

RADIOLOGY HOT LIST

- Benign bony lesions are classically well defined (a 'narrow zone of transition'). They typically expand the bone (implying slow growth) rather than destroying it. There should be no associated aggressive periosteal reaction or soft tissue mass present.
- The proximal femur is a typical location for fibrous dysplasia, where it may cause modelling deformities leading to a 'shepherd's-crook' appearance. The lesion may have an internal ground-glass (hazy) appearance.
- Other bones affected by fibrous dysplasia include the skull and facial bones (typically sclerotic lesions), ribs and pelvis.

CLINICAL HOT LIST

- Fibrous dysplasia is a developmental anomaly of the mesenchymal precursor of bone, causing areas of immature collagen matrix with small irregular bony trabeculae within the medullary cavity.
- Fibrous dysplasia may be monostotic (70%, one bone affected, later presentation) or polyostotic (30%, multiple bones involved, often unilateral, presentation in childhood).
- Polyostotic fibrous dysplasia is associated with McCune–Albright syndrome, which occurs predominantly in females. There is precocious puberty, and 'coast of Maine' café-au-lait spots are seen on the back, trunk, shoulders, and buttocks.
- The bone lesions may be asymptomatic or cause pain and limp. First presentation may be with a pathological fracture.

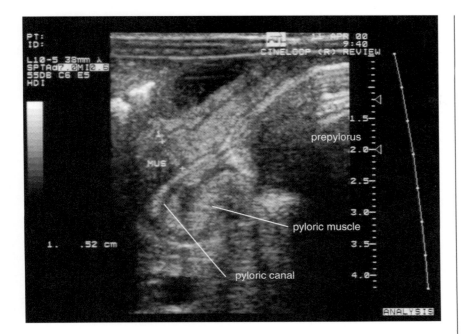

This 6 week old boy was admitted with vomiting after feeds and weight loss. On examination, he was hungry and wasted. Visible peristalsis was observed.

1. What examination has been performed?
2. What is the most likely diagnosis?

ANSWERS

1. Abdominal ultrasound to assess the pylorus.
2. Hypertrophic pyloric stenosis.

RADIOLOGY HOT LIST

- Ultrasound is the investigation of choice, though the diagnosis is often made clinically.
- The findings are of an enlarged pylorus, >17 mm in longitudinal section, or >13 mm in transverse section. The pyloric muscle thickness is >4 mm.
- The area should be scanned continuously during a feed to demonstrate lack of opening of the pyloric canal with exaggerated peristalsis. This is the most sensitive imaging finding for this condition.
- A barium meal may show shouldering of the antrum with elongation and narrowing of the pyloric canal ('string sign').

CLINICAL HOT LIST

- The condition is due to idiopathic hypertrophy of the circular muscle of the pylorus.
- It classically affects firstborn males at 2–8 weeks of life.
- Presentation is with non-bilious projectile vomiting, inadequate weight gain and a hungry baby.
- Clinical examination of the abdomen may demonstrate visible peristalsis, and the enlarged pylorus may be felt as a palpable 'olive-shaped' mass.
- Surgical pyloromyotomy is curative.

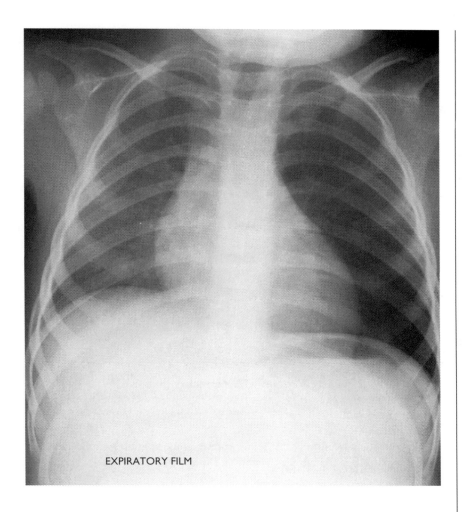

EXPIRATORY FILM

This 3 year old boy was seen in A&E with sudden onset of coughing and acute respiratory distress.

1. What does the chest radiograph show?
2. What is the diagnosis?

ANSWERS

1. The left lung is of greater volume and is hyperlucent compared to the right. As the film is deliberately taken in expiration, this implies air trapping on the left. The normal right lung is smaller because it is an expiratory film. (Don't get caught out — it can be difficult to tell which side is abnormal.)
2. Inhaled foreign body in the left main bronchus (a peanut).

RADIOLOGY HOT LIST

- The normal cross-sectional diameter of the airway increases in inspiration and decreases in expiration. Foreign bodies can cause three radiological appearances according to their size:

Small (<%)	normal CXR, no obstruction to air flow
Intermediate (80%)	hyperinflation due to air trapping. Occlusion occurs in expiration only, due to normal decrease in bronchial diameter around the foreign body
Large (20%)	distal consolidation and atelectasis due to complete obstruction of airway

- Children unable to cooperate with expiratory films can be assessed for air trapping with screening or decubitus views (lying on suspect side, which would normally reduce in volume but remains hyperinflated due to presence of foreign body).
- Pneumomediastinum and pneumothorax are potential complications.
- Foreign bodies are often not radio–opaque!

CLINICAL HOT LIST

- Usually occurs in children under 4 years (M > F).
- They commonly present with sudden choking, cough and wheeze, which may subsequently settle. Delayed presentation occurs in up to 30%.
- The treatment of choice is bronchoscopic removal of the foreign body.

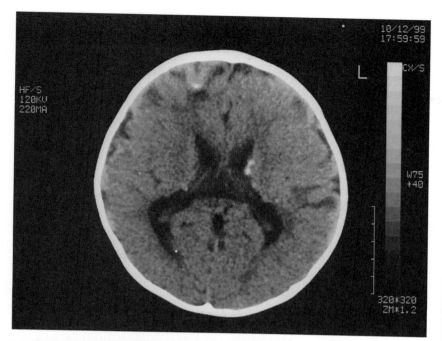

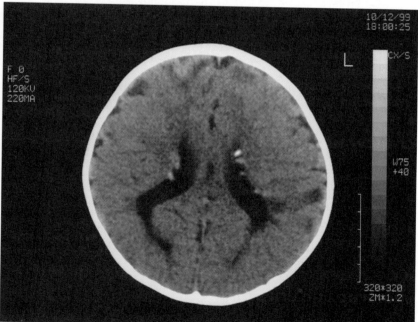

A 3 month old girl presented with a history of frequent seizures. Investigations included a CT scan of the brain.

1. What abnormalities are present on the non–enhanced scan?
2. What is the diagnosis?

ANSWERS

1. There are multiple calcified subependymal nodules with a 'candle drippings' appearance along the lining of the lateral ventricles. There are several low-attenuation areas in the cerebral cortex which represent cortical tubers, one of which is calcified.
2. Tuberous sclerosis.

RADIOLOGICAL HOT LIST

- The typical findings in tuberous sclerosis are subependymal hamartomas protruding into the lateral ventricles. These calcify with increasing age.
- Cortical or subcortical hamartomas (tubers) are seen on CT as hypodense lesions (typically non-calcified).
- 5–15% will develop a giant cell astrocytoma at the foramen of Munro, usually causing hydrocephalus.
- Other causes of intracerebral calcification at this age include intrauterine cytomegalovirus and toxoplasmosis infection. These will not show the typical subependymal location.

CLINICAL HOT LIST

- Tuberous sclerosis is an autosomal dominant condition. 50% result from spontaneous mutation.
- Cardinal features include multiple facial angiofibromas (adenoma sebaceum), subungual fibromas, retinal hamartomas and cortical tubers.
- Cutaneous features include white macules, which fluoresce under Woods light, and shagreen patches. Cardiac rhabdomyomas and renal tumours (angiomyofibromas and renal cysts) may occur.
- Seizures are the most common presenting symptom (seen in up to 90%). Infants may present with infantile spasms. Early seizures correlate with significant learning difficulties.

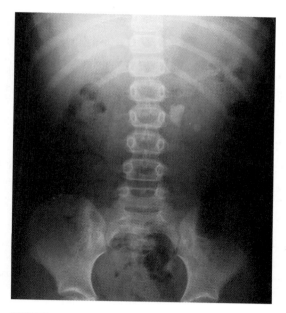

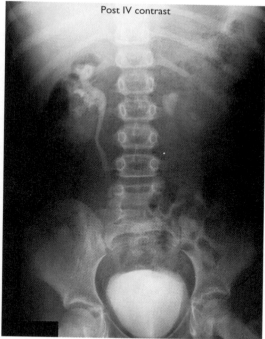

Post IV contrast

This 6 year old boy has left flank pain and haematuria.

1. What abnormalities are seen on the plain film and intravenous urogram (IVU)?
2. What is the diagnosis?

ANSWERS

1. On the plain film there are opacities projected over the left renal hilum and the lower pole of the left kidney. On the IVU, the right kidney excretes normally. No contrast is seen in the left pelvicalyceal system.
2. Left staghorn calculus with an obstructed kidney. Further calculus in the left lower pole.

RADIOLOGY HOT LIST

- IVUs are performed infrequently in children (ultrasound and nuclear medicine are the investigations of choice) but are useful in cases of renal stones.
- Small renal calculi may be difficult to see on ultrasound but 90% of renal calculi are visible on the plain film.
- Always assess the preliminary abdominal X-ray for evidence of renal tract calcification, which may be obscured by contrast.
- Obstruction results in delayed or absent excretion of contrast on the affected side.

CLINICAL HOT LIST

- Renal calculi are rare in children: the majority are related to stasis secondary to obstruction, or infection. Patients with congenital abnormalities such as bladder diverticulum, horseshoe kidney and medullary sponge kidney have an increased incidence.
- 10% of calculi are due to metabolic causes:

Stone type	Cause
Calcium stones	hypercalcuria, hypercalcaemia secondary to hyperpara-thyroidism, excess vitamin D
Cystine stones	cystinuria with renal tubular defect of amino acid transport
Oxalate stones	primary hyperoxaluria, or secondary to small bowel disease and disordered absorption, e.g. Crohn's, post-surgical
Uric acid stones	induction therapy for leukaemia

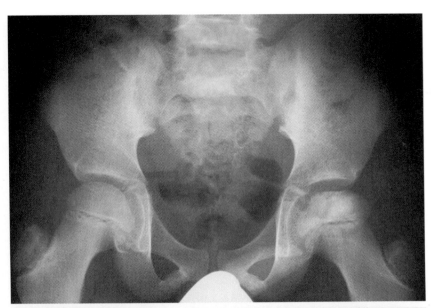

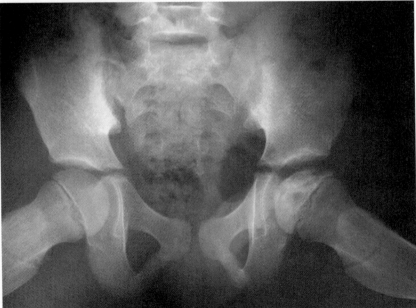

This 6 year old boy presented to his GP with a 2 week history of left groin pain and a limp.

AP and frog-lateral pelvic X-rays were obtained.

1. What do they show?
2. What is the diagnosis?
3. What are the sequelae if untreated?

ANSWERS

1. There is flattening and sclerosis of the left femoral capital epiphysis with subchondral fissures.
2. Perthes disease (idiopathic avascular necrosis of the femoral head).
3. Abnormal bony remodelling with severe degenerative joint disease in early adulthood.

RADIOLOGY HOT LIST

- In the early phase the plain film is normal, but MRI will show bone marrow changes and a bone scan may show a focal photopenic defect.
- Plain film changes reflect the healing process.
- A frog-lateral X-ray may be more sensitive than the AP view of the pelvis in demonstrating early changes.

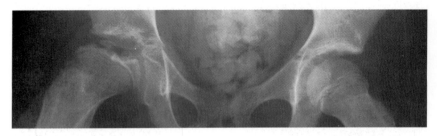

Late changes include a flattened misshapen femoral head with a short widened femoral neck.

- Consider underlying pathology such as sickle cell disease, steroid therapy, and Gaucher's disease. Avascular necrosis can also occur secondary to trauma, infection, surgery and traction.

CLINICAL HOT LIST

- Idiopathic avascular necrosis of the femoral head in childhood is due to interruption of the blood supply to the femoral epiphysis.
- It most commonly occurs in boys (4:1) aged between 4 and 10 years, and is bilateral in 10%.
- Clinical symptoms are gradual in onset with no recalled history of trauma. It may present with groin pain, limp, or limited hip movement.
- Treatment may include rest, traction, abduction bracing and osteotomy.

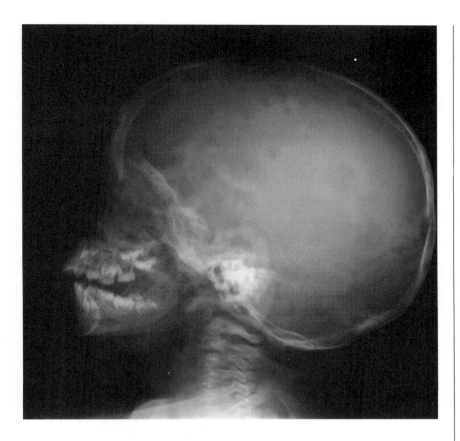

1. What abnormality is demonstrated on this lateral skull X-ray?
2. What is the most likely diagnosis?
3. What is the differential diagnosis?

ANSWERS

1. Well-defined, rounded lucent lesions are seen throughout the skull.
2. Langerhans' cell histiocytosis.
3. Bone metastases, most commonly from neuroblastoma or leukaemia.

RADIOLOGY HOT LIST

- The skull is the most common site for bone involvement in Langerhans' cell histiocytosis.
- The lesions are usually well defined and may have a sclerotic rim, giving a 'bevelled' edge appearance.
- The spine and ribs are also commonly involved. Radiological findings in the spine include lytic lesions and vertebral collapse (vertebra plana).

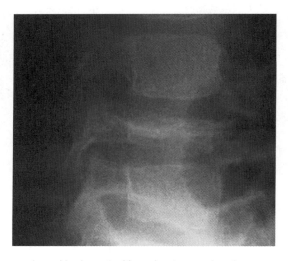

Lateral lumbar spine X-ray showing vertebra plana.

- Lytic lesions and periosteal reactions may be seen in the long bones.
- Extraskeletal disease may manifest radiologically as pulmonary interstitial infiltrates and pneumothorax.

CLINICAL HOT LIST

- Langerhans' cell histiocytosis is a disease of unknown aetiology with abnormal proliferation of phagocytic histiocytes.
- There may be multisystem involvement, and the clinical course can vary from relatively benign to highly malignant and fatal.
- The disease process may involve skin, lungs, bone marrow, lympho-reticular system (lymphadenopathy and hepatosplenomegaly), bone and the pituitary (diabetes insipidus).
- The treatment may include chemotherapy and radiotherapy.

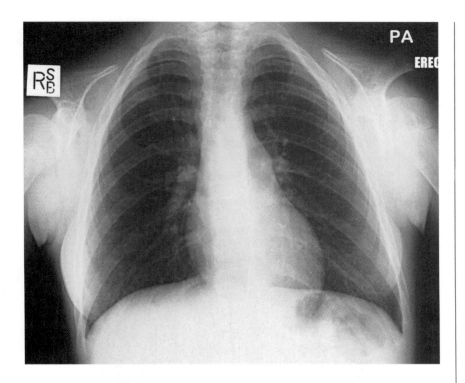

This 12 year old girl had a chest infection when this X-ray was taken.

1. What abnormalities are seen on the chest X-ray?
2. What is the diagnosis?

ANSWERS

1. The clavicles are absent. The lungs are clear .
2. Cleidocranial dysostosis.

RADIOLOGY HOT LIST

- The clavicles may be hypoplastic or absent (10%).
- The chest may be narrow or bell shaped, with supernumerary ribs.
- The skull typically shows deficient ossification, widened sutures and fontanelles, and Wormian bones (small accessory bones within the sutures).

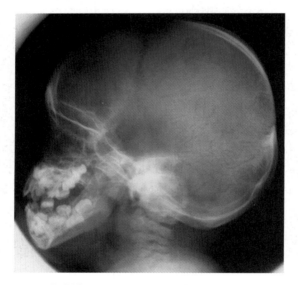

Skull X-ray showing multiple Wormian bones.

CLINICAL HOT LIST

- Autosomal dominant disease with delayed/defective ossification of mid-line structures (particularly membranous bone).
- Characteristic features:

Face	hypoplastic maxilla, broad depressed bridge of nose, hypertelorism
Teeth	delayed and abnormal dentition, malocclusion
Pelvis	hypoplastic pubic rami, pubic diastasis
Hands	long second metacarpal
Other features	short stature, coxa vara

- Management requires orthopaedic and dental input.

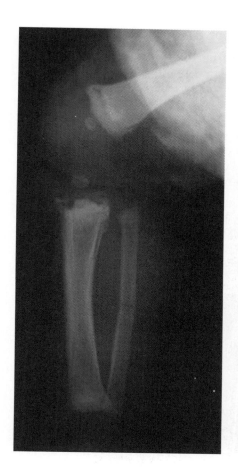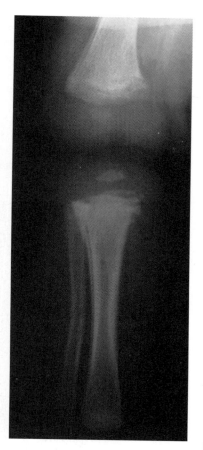

This 3 month old baby presented to A&E with a history of inconsolable crying. On examination, he was not moving his right leg, which appeared swollen. His mother attributed this to an injury earlier in the week while changing his nappy.

1. What abnormality is seen on the AP and lateral views of the right leg?
2. What is the diagnosis?

ANSWERS

1. There are metaphyseal fractures of the distal right femur and proximal right tibia, with an exuberant callus response and periosteal reactions along the shaft of both bones. There is a more recent fracture involving the midshaft of the right fibula.
2. Non–accidental injury.

RADIOLOGY HOT LIST

Radiological features in long bones suggestive of NAI:

● Fractures of different ages (new fracture/periosteal reaction/mature callus formation).
● Metaphyseal fractures ('bucket-handle' or 'corner-chip') are pathognomic of non–accidental injury. These may be subtle and meticulous radiography is required.

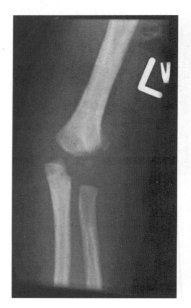 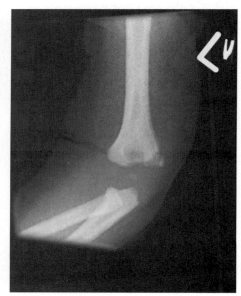

Examples of metaphyseal fractures.

● Solitary transverse or spiral fractures are much more common in NAI and the history is crucial in assessing the appropriateness of the injury.
● A fracture in a non-ambulant child should always be regarded with suspicion.
● Exaggerated callus formation is due to repetitive injury and/or a lack of treatment/immobilisation.
● WARNING: the initial plain film may be normal – late films are essential if NAI is suspected. Bone scan may show abnormalities before the plain films.

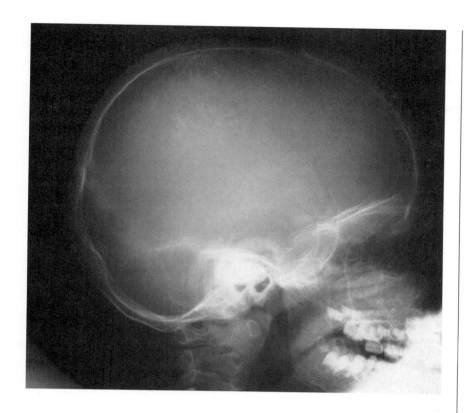

This 8 year old Greek girl has chronic anaemia.

1. What does the lateral skull radiograph show?
2. What is the diagnosis?

ANSWERS

1. There is skull vault thickening, with widening of the diploic space and thinning of the cortical margins of the inner and outer tables of the skull. The paranasal air sinuses and mastoid air cells are radio-opaque.
2. β-Thalassaemia

RADIOLOGY HOT LIST

- Skull vault thickening occurs due to marrow hyperplasia (extramedullary haemopoiesis). The cortex of the inner and outer tables is progressively thinned, and nearly invisible – if only the coarsened vertical trabeculations are seen, this leads to a 'hair-on-end' appearance.
- Involvement of the facial bones causes non-pneumatisation of the paranasal air sinuses and mastoid air cells.
- The small bones of the hands and feet may show modelling deformities, cortical thinning and a coarsened trabecular pattern.
- Extramedullary haemopoiesis may cause a paravertebral mass on the chest X-ray.

CLINICAL HOT LIST

- β-Thalassaemia is a haemoglobinopathy caused by abnormal β globin chain synthesis. It is commonly found in people of Mediterranean and Asian descent.
- It presents in the first year of life (when Hb A replaces Hb F). Features include anaemia, hepatosplenomegaly, recurrent fever and failure to thrive.
- Skeletal deformities may be prevented by a regular transfusion programme. Haemosiderosis may occur due to frequent transfusions and increased iron absorption. It can be prevented by iron chelation with desferrioxamine.
- Splenectomy may be required when splenomegaly and increasing transfusion requirements become problematical.
- Bone marrow transplantation is potentially curative.

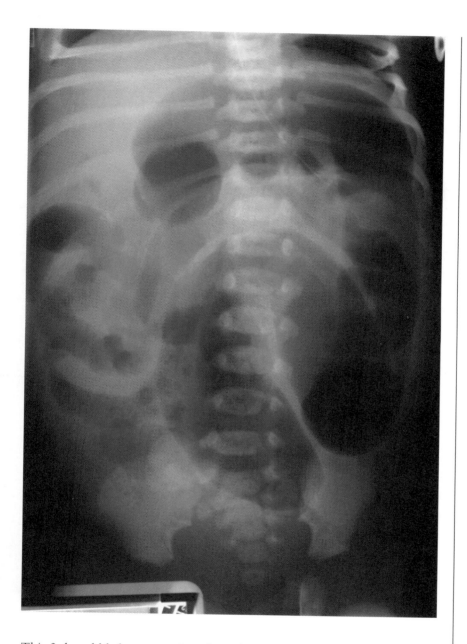

This 3 day old baby was reviewed on the postnatal ward for failure to pass meconium. On examination the abdomen was distended with palpable bowel loops, and the anus appeared patent.

1. What two abnormalities are seen on the plain abdominal X-ray?
2. What is the most likely diagnosis?
3. What is the differential diagnosis?

ANSWERS

1. There are dilated loops of small and large bowel within the abdomen. The sigmoid colon appears dilated. No gas is seen in the rectum.
2. Hirschsprung's disease.
3. The differential diagnosis of neonatal large bowel obstruction is functional immaturity (including meconium plug syndrome) and anorectal atresia.

RADIOLOGY HOT LIST

- Differentiating between small and large bowel obstruction is difficult in neonates. Look for anatomical location of bowel loops; if central, they are more likely to be small bowel.
- A contrast enema will differentiate between the major causes of low bowel obstruction: Hirschsprung's, atresia, meconium ileus, functional motility disorders (meconium plug syndrome).
- A contrast enema in Hirschsprung's disease may delineate the transition zone between normal (innervated) dilated colon and the narrowed segment of aganglionic bowel. This is usually in the rectosigmoid region.

CLINICAL HOT LIST

- Pathology: absent ganglia in both myenteric plexi (Auerbach and Meissner). The distribution is from the anus proximally, explained by a failure of caudal migration of neural crest cells.
- Presentation varies with length of affected bowel: 70% short segment, 25% long segment, 5% total colon (short segment may present as chronic constipation in the older child).
- **The diagnosis is made by rectal biopsy.** Management is surgical: either primary pull through, or colostomy and delayed definitive procedure.
- 5% also have Down's syndrome.
- Complications include necrotising enterocolitis (the risk persists even after surgery), perforation and failure to thrive.

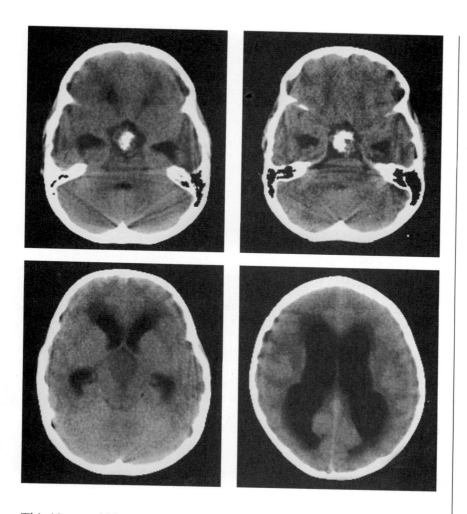

This 10 year old boy was being investigated for headaches. On examination he had a bitemporal hemianopia.

1. Describe two radiological abnormalities seen on the non-enhanced CT scan.
2. What is the diagnosis?

ANSWERS

1. There is a densely calcified suprasellar mass present. There is dilatation of the lateral ventricles (obstructive hydrocephalus). Periventricular low attenuation indicates acute hydrocephalus requiring urgent shunting.
2. Craniopharyngioma.

RADIOLOGY HOT LIST

- Skull X-rays may be normal, or show an enlarged or eroded pituitary fossa with associated calcification.
- CT shows a cystic (75%) or mixed solid/cystic suprasellar mass, which is calcified in 70%. Large lesions may cause obstructive hydrocephalus.
- MRI is performed to assess local spread, e.g. involvement of optic chiasm and extension to hypothalamus.

CLINICAL HOT LIST

- Craniopharyngiomas are the commonest cause of a childhood suprasellar mass (median age of presentation 8 years).
- Presenting features include signs of raised intracranial pressure secondary to obstructive hydrocephalus, and visual field defects (classically bitemporal hemianopia).
- Endocrine dysfunction may occur as a result of abnormal levels of growth hormone, ACTH, TSH, TRH and ADH. The child may present with growth retardation or diabetes insipidus.
- Management is surgical resection, radiotherapy and endocrine replacement therapy.

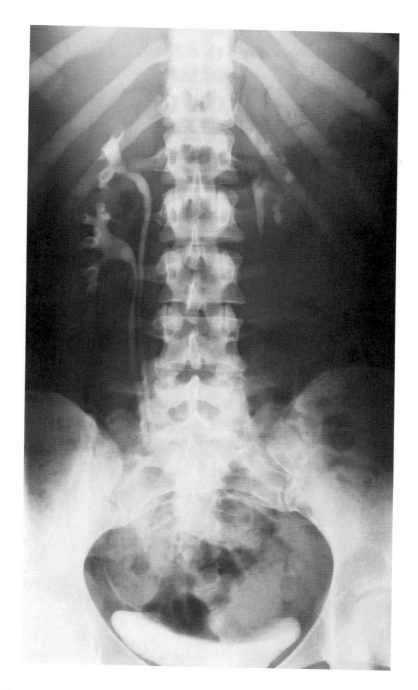

This teenage girl complained of continuous incontinence, present since birth. An intravenous urogram (IVU) was performed.

1. What does the study show?
2. What is the diagnosis?

ANSWERS

1. There is a duplex system on the right side with two non-dilated ureters. The left kidney is small.
2. Duplex right kidney. The presence of continuous incontinence suggests that the upper moeity ureter inserts in an extravesical location. (The scarred left kidney is due to severe reflux nephropathy on this side.)

RADIOLOGY HOT LIST

- An IVU is rarely indicated in children. However, it demonstrates the renal tract anatomy when there is suspicion of a duplex collecting system. The ureters may unite or have separate insertions.
- Classically the upper moiety has an ectopic insertion, usually into the bladder. Insertion into the bladder neck, urethra or vagina results in incontinence. The ectopic insertion makes the upper moiety prone to obstruction.
- There may be an associated ureterocele (seen as a filling defect in the bladder).
- Ultrasound can demonstrate many of these features including the obstructed upper moiety and dilated ureter. Always consider the diagnosis where there is a 'cystic' lesion arising from the upper pole.
- The lower moiety may have a 'drooping flower' appearance on IVU (obstructed upper moiety displacing middle and lower pole calyces downward) and is prone to vesicoureteric reflux and renal scarring.

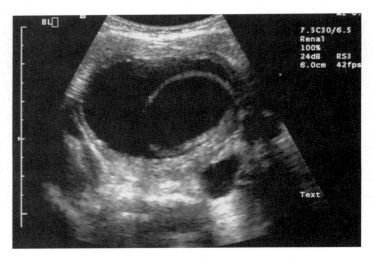

Ultrasound image of an ureterocele within the bladder.

CLINICAL HOT LIST

- Complete duplication occurs in 0.5–10% of livebirths, F > M, and is bilateral in 15–40%.

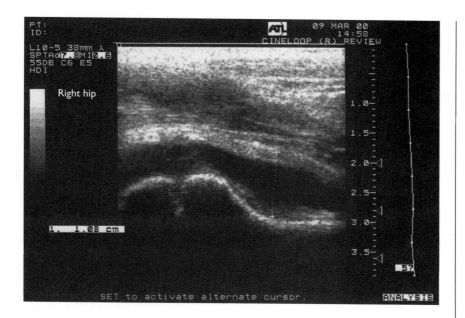

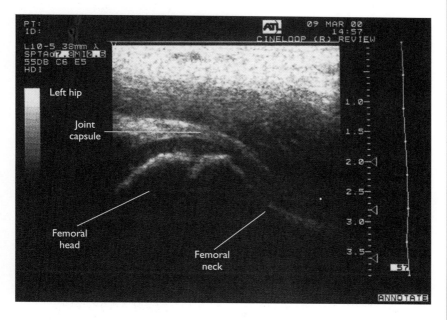

This 4 year old boy presented to the GP with a 3 day history of fever and coryzal symptoms, and a 1 day history of right-sided limp. An ultrasound examination of his hips was performed.

1. What does the ultrasound show?
2. What is the most likely diagnosis?

ANSWERS

1. There is a joint effusion present in the right hip. The joint capsule is distended anteriorly with anechoic fluid lying between the capsule and the femoral neck. The left hip joint is normal.
2. Transient synovititis of the right hip (irritable hip), though a septic arthritis will need to be excluded.

RADIOLOGY HOT LIST

- Ultrasound is the examination of choice for the detection of a joint effusion. Comparison can be made between the normal and affected side. It will allow aspiration of fluid if a septic arthritis needs to be excluded.
- Radiological evaluation of childhood limp should include an X-ray of the pelvis to look for bony pathology. Plain films are relatively insensitive at detecting effusions, but large effusions may cause a relative increase in the medial joint space (asymmetry of greater than 2 mm is pathological).

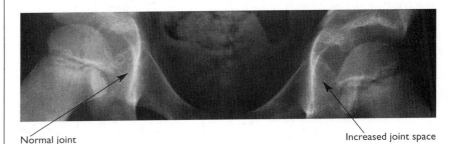

Normal joint   Increased joint space

CLINICAL HOT LIST

- Irritable hip occurs most commonly in boys aged 3–10 years. It usually follows a viral infection, presenting with sudden onset of hip pain and a low-grade pyrexia. It is managed conservatively, with bed rest and analgesia.
- The primary differential diagnosis is septic arthritis, when the serum inflammatory markers are usually raised. However the definitive test remains microbiological analysis of aspirated joint fluid.
- Causes of a joint effusion include transient synovitis, septic arthritis, trauma, juvenile idiopathic arthritis, and early Perthes disease.
- Hip pathology may present with referred knee pain.

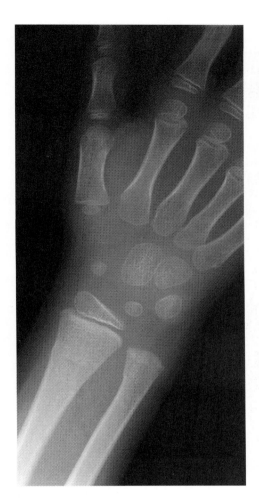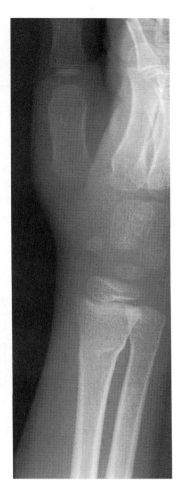

This 5 year old boy attended A&E after a fall whilst playing.

1. What abnormality is seen on the plain radiograph of the right wrist?
2. What is the diagnosis?

ANSWERS

1. There is buckling of the cortex of the distal radius and ulna with a faint transverse lucency seen in the distal radius.
2. Torus fractures of the distal radius and ulna.

RADIOLOGY HOT LIST

- The cortex of a bone is normally a smooth unbroken line.
- Impaction results in cortical buckling and a torus fracture (torus is derived from the Latin word meaning protruberance or bulge).
- A greenstick fracture (less common) occurs if the bone is angulated beyond its capacity for bending, leading to a fracture on the convex side of the bend. Muscular spasm may then hold the fracture open at this 'hinge' point.

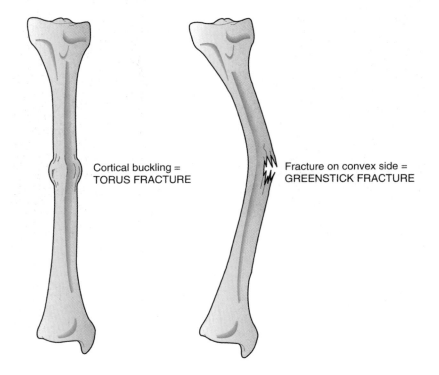

Cortical buckling =
TORUS FRACTURE

Fracture on convex side =
GREENSTICK FRACTURE

CLINICAL HOT LIST

- Torus fractures are treated with immobilisation and pain relief.
- Greenstick fractures with pronounced angulation may require reduction and correct positioning prior to immobilisation and healing.

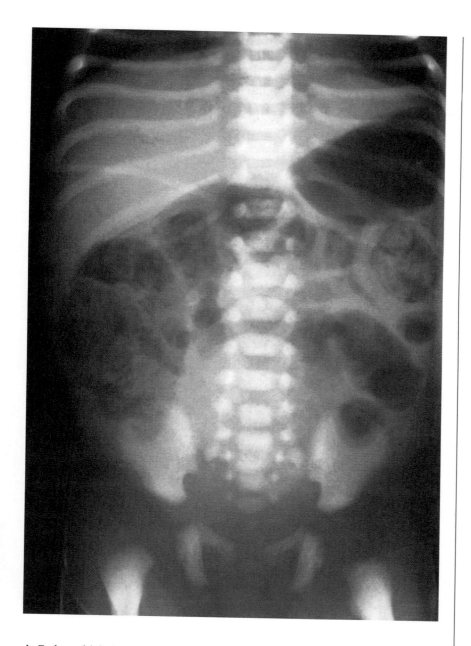

A 7 day old baby, born at 29 weeks' gestation, is noted to be pale and lethargic on the neonatal unit.

1. What radiological sign is seen on the plain abdominal radiograph?
2. What is the diagnosis?
3. Give four possible risk factors for this condition.

ANSWERS

1. There are linear lucencies within the bowel wall, representing intramural gas (pneumatosis intestinalis). There is no evidence of perforation, or gas within the portal venous system.
2. Necrotising enterocolitis (NEC).
3. Risk factors include prematurity, intrauterine growth retardation, perinatal asphyxia, hypoxia and shock, sepsis, polycythaemia, umbilical catheterisation and hypertonic feeds.

RADIOLOGY HOT LIST

- The initial plain film may be normal. Early radiological signs include dilated loops of bowel and bowel wall thickening. The colon and terminal ileum are most commonly affected.
- Intramural gas is characteristic of NEC, and may appear as linear lucencies or 'foamy' collections of gas.
- Search for free air, which may appear as a central lucency overlying the abdomen (as the baby is supine), or outlining the falciform ligament (which appears as an opaque line in the midline or right upper quadrant).
- Look for portal venous gas (linear lucencies within the liver which extend peripherally).

CLINICAL HOT LIST

- It is primarily a condition of preterm and low birthweight babies whose immature gut is vulnerable to a variety of insults, which manifest as NEC.
- Cardinal mechanisms are gut hypoperfusion and ischaemia, though an infective process is also implicated.
- Clinical presentation ranges from systemic features (lethargy, hypotonia, shock and apnoea) to abdominal distension, bilious vomiting and rectal bleeding.
- Management of NEC is usually conservative (resuscitation, systemic support, total parenteral nutrition and antibiotics). Surgical intervention may be required for perforation or failure of medical management.
- Late complications include intestinal stricture (20%) and short gut syndrome (post-surgical resection).

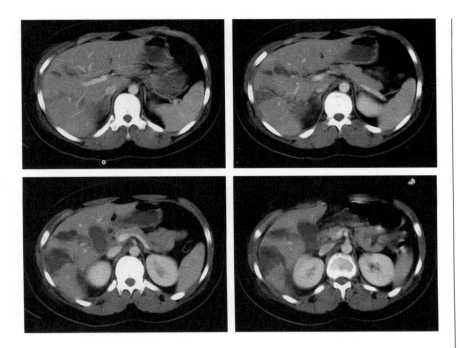

This 13 year old boy was involved in a road traffic accident, and complained of right upper quadrant pain.

1. What does the contrast-enhanced CT scan of the abdomen show?
2. What is the diagnosis?

ANSWERS

1. There are multiple, irregular, low-attenuation areas within the right lobe of the liver. The intrahepatic vessels are normally opacified. No free fluid is present. The intra-abdominal appearances are otherwise normal.
2. Multiple liver lacerations with haematomas secondary to blunt trauma.

RADIOLOGY HOT LIST

- Liver lacerations are typically branching or rounded low attentuation areas.
- Haematomas usually appear as poorly defined areas of low attenuation. High attenuation areas may represent active haemorrhage.
- A subcapsular haematoma usually has a lenticular or crescent-shaped configuration.
- Look for free fluid (haemoperitoneum) and other visceral injuries. There is an associated splenic injury in 45%.

CLINICAL HOT LIST

- The liver is the second most frequently injured intra-abdominal viscus (after the spleen) in blunt trauma. The right lobe is most commonly affected.
- Liver trauma is usually managed conservatively (in >90% children). Embolisation or surgery is indicated for continued bleeding.
- Complications occur in up to 20% (delayed rupture, haemobilia, infected haematoma, arteriovenous fistula).

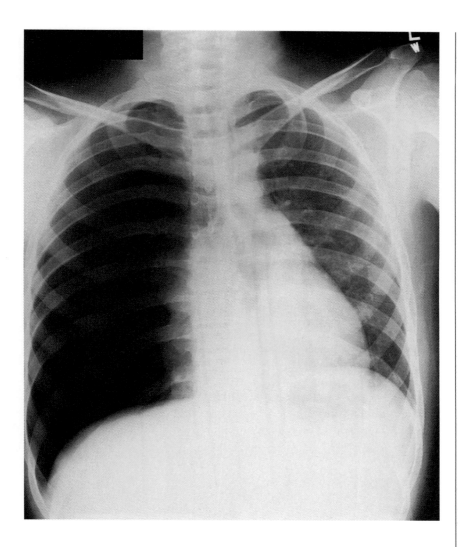

This 16 year old boy presented to A&E with an acute onset of dyspnoea and pleuritic chest pain.

1. What does the chest X-ray show?
2. What is the diagnosis?

ANSWERS

1. The right hemithorax is hyperlucent with complete absence of pulmonary markings. The right hemidiaphragm is depressed and the mediastinum is displaced to the left.
2. Right tension pneumothorax.

RADIOLOGY HOT LIST

- Always assess the pulmonary vascularity when considering unequal lucency on the CXR – is it normal, reduced (implying abnormal lung), or absent (pneumothorax)?
- Look for a free lung edge. Mediastinal shift and/or a depressed diaphragm indicate the presence of a tension pneumothorax.
- Other causes of a unilateral hyperlucent hemithorax include patient rotation, air trapping (e.g. secondary to foreign body, congenital lobar emphysema), reduced pulmonary perfusion, and chest wall abnormalities.

CLINICAL HOT LIST

- Childhood pneumothorax is associated with trauma, asthma, cystic fibrosis, pulmonary infections (including TB), Marfan's syndrome and mechanical ventilation.
- Treatment options include observation, simple aspiration and chest drain insertion. The choice will depend on clinical presentation and severity.
- Life-threatening tension pneumothorax needs immediate intervention: do not wait for an X-ray!

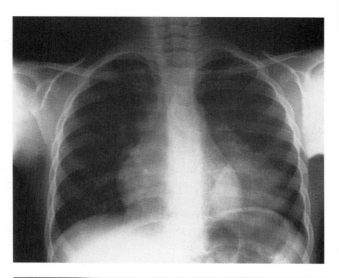

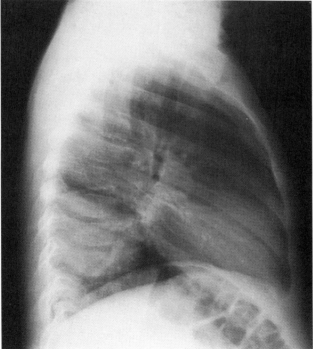

A 3 year old girl was admitted via A&E with fever and cough. On examination she is pyrexial, with tachypnoea and tachycardia.

1. What abnormality is seen on the AP and lateral CXR?
2. What is the most likely diagnosis?

ANSWERS

1. There is a rounded opacity in the left lower lobe, which is intra-pulmonary, and clearly separated from the spine. There is no air–fluid level or rib erosion.
2. Left lower lobe round pneumonia.

RADIOLOGY HOT LIST

- Round pneumonia is the most common cause of an apparent mass lesion in the paediatric chest. In the appropriate clinical setting a follow-up chest X-ray after antibiotic therapy is the most pragmatic approach. With time, the initially round pneumonia develops into a more typical consolidation before eventual resolution.
- The lesion is clearly not paravertebral, making neurogenic tumours, a paraspinal abscess or extramedullary haematopoiesis unlikely.
- Other causes of solitary lung nodules:

Congenital	bronchogenic cyst, lung sequestration, arteriovenous malformation, bronchial atresia
Infection	abscess, granuloma
Tumour	primary lung tumour: primitive neuroectodermal tumour (PNET), pulmonary blastoma, metastases (e.g. Wilm's tumour)

CLINICAL HOT LIST

- Round pneumonia is usually seen in the early consolidative phase of pneumococcal pneumonia.

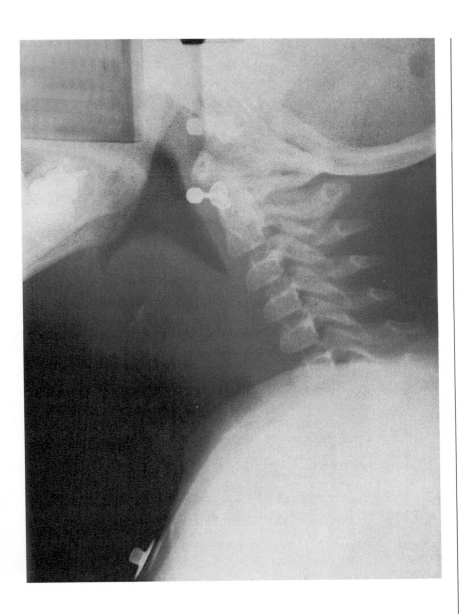

A 4 year old girl has a fever and sore throat. On examination she is pyrexial (40°C) and drooling.

1. What abnormality does the lateral X-ray of the neck show?
2. What is the diagnosis?

ANSWERS

1. The epiglottis is enlarged and indistinct and encroaches on the pharynx. The upper airway is distended.
2. Acute epiglottitis.

RADIOLOGY HOT LIST

- Epiglottitis is a clinical diagnosis and a paediatric emergency. Radiographs are not required to make the diagnosis! If X-rays are performed, the child must be accompanied by a physician skilled in managing a paediatric airway – the risk of complete airway obstruction is very real.
- The normal epiglottis has a well-defined slender shape – in acute epiglottitis this shape is lost as the epiglottis becomes swollen, with swelling of the adjacent aryepiglottic folds, leading to airway obstruction.

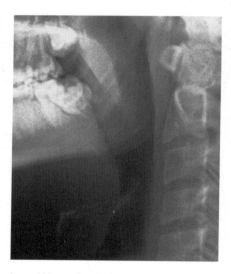

Lateral X-ray of neck showing normal epiglottis.

- The upper airway may be distended (airway obstruction) and the neck held in extension (to keep airway patent).

CLINICAL HOT LIST

- It is due to a severe bacterial infection, usually occurring in 2 to 7 year olds. It is now rare due to the *Haemophilus influenzae B* vaccination.
- Clinical presentation: sudden onset of sore throat and dysphagia, progressing to signs of upper airway obstruction in a febrile toxic child.
- No investigations are necessary prior to diagnostic laryngoscopy. Intubation may be required. This must be undertaken in a controlled manner in theatre with the most experienced anaesthetist available.
- Further management includes intravenous antibiotics and intensive care.

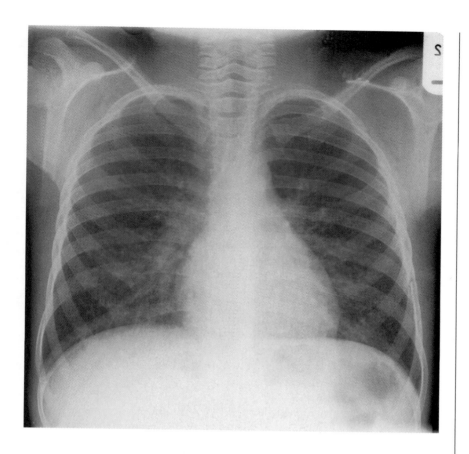

This 6 year old HIV-positive boy has a cough.

1. What does the chest radiograph show?
2. What is the diagnosis?

ANSWERS

1. There is fine reticular nodular shadowing throughout the lungs, more prominent at the bases. There is no apparent mediastinal lymphadenopathy.
2. Lymphoid interstitial pneumonitis (LIP).

RADIOLOGY HOT LIST

- The appearances are variable, but there is usually reticular nodular shadowing (opacities up to 5 mm) present. This may progress to areas of more confluent air space shadowing. The chest X-ray may be normal.
- High-resolution CT chest scans may show extensive bronchovascular micronodules and ground-glass attenuation.
- These appearances may be mimicked by infection and a lung biopsy may be required to make the diagnosis.

CLINICAL HOT LIST

- It is a lymphoproliferative disorder characterised by diffuse lymphocytic infiltration of the pulmonary interstitium, possibly secondary to direct pulmonary HIV infection.
- It is indicative of AIDS when present in children (much less common in HIV positive adults), and is present in 55% of children with AIDS who have pulmonary disease.
- It is a slowly progressive disorder with dyspnoea, dry cough, fever, weight loss, generalised lymphadenopathy and hepatosplenomegaly. It is associated with bilateral chronic parotitis.
- It has a variable clinical course, but overall these children develop fewer opportunistic infections.

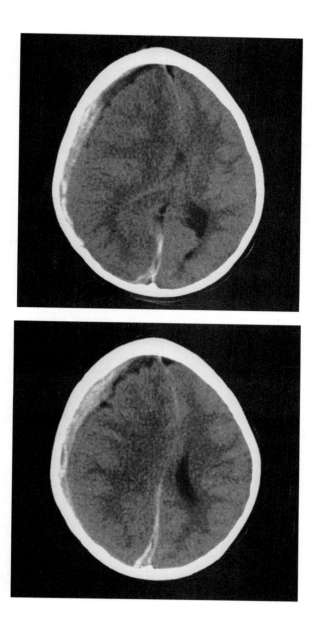

This 3 year old girl was brought to A&E after a sudden collapse. On examination she was unresponsive to pain with bradycardia.

1. Name three abnormalities seen on the non-enhanced CT scan of the head.
2. What is the diagnosis?
3. What is the most likely underlying cause?

ANSWERS

1. There is midline shift and effacement of the right lateral ventricle. There is a right subdural collection with areas of high and low attenuation within it. A further high attenuation subdural collection is seen posteriorly, along the interhemispheric fissure, adjacent to the falx cerebri.
2. Acute on chronic right subdural haematoma and an acute inter-hemispheric fissure subdural haematoma.
3. Non-accidental injury (NAI).

RADIOLOGY HOT LIST

- Subdural collections appear as crescent shaped, often extending widely across the convexity of a cerebral hemisphere.
- Fresh blood appears initially as high density, becomes isodense with brain after 7–10 days, and low density after 3–4 weeks.
- Features of subdural haematomas that are suspicious for NAI:
  —Subdural haematoma with no associated skull fracture implying shaking injury.
  —Bilateral subdurals.
  —Subdurals of different ages (areas of high and low attenuation).
  —Acute interhemispheric fissure subdural or falx haemorrhage (bright irregularly thickened falx).
  —Subdurals in the presence of retinal haemorrhages, implying acceleration/deceleration force.

CLINICAL HOT LIST

	Acute subdural	Chronic subdural
Time of injury	< 3 days	> 3 weeks
Presentation	Shock, raised intracranial pressure, cerebral oedema	Insidious, few clinical signs, no raised intracranial pressure
Outcome	50% mortality. Survivors have high risk of severe neurological deficit	80% full recovery

- Subdural haematoma is uncommon in accidental head injury but usually present in most fatal head injuries caused by non-accidental injury.
- The mechanism of injury is rotation of the brain within the fixed cranial vault and dura, causing tearing of the bridging veins. Associated retinal haemorrhages are present in up to 70%.
- Neurosurgical consultation is mandatory, with intensive care management of raised intracranial pressure (in an acute presentation).
- All cases of suspected NAI require detailed clinical examination, documentation of all injuries, fundoscopy, skeletal survey and involvement of the child protection team.

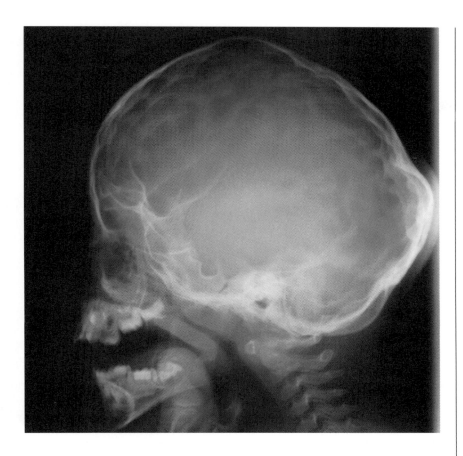

This 2 year old boy has developmental delay.

1. What does the lateral skull X-ray show?
2. What is the diagnosis?

ANSWERS

1. The skull is microcephalic and has an abnormal shape. The normal sagittal, coronal and lambdoid sutures are obliterated (fused). There is a 'copper-beaten' appearance to the skull (due to prominent convolutional markings on the inner table).
2. Craniosynostosis with raised intracranial pressure.

RADIOLOGY HOT LIST

- Craniosynostosis refers to premature closure of one or more skull sutures, leading to an abnormally shaped skull.
- Involvement of individual sutures gives rise to characteristic deformities, e.g. premature fusion of the sagittal suture results in scaphocephaly.
- If all three sutures are involved raised intracranial pressure may result, manifesting as the 'copper-beaten' skull. (This appearance can be normal before the age of 6 months.)

CLINICAL HOT LIST

- Craniosynostosis may be primary or secondary.

Causes of secondary craniosynostosis	Examples
Syndromes (associated with syndactyly and polysyndactyly)	Apert, Carpenter, Crouzon, Pfieffer, clover leaf skull
Haematological	sickle cell anaemia, thalassaemia
Metabolic	rickets, hypercalcaemia, hyperthyroidism
Bone dysplasia	hypophosphatasia, achondroplasia, metaphyseal dysplasia
Microcephaly	brain atrophy/dysgenesis
Postsurgical	post-shunting procedures

- Presentation may be with an abnormal head shape, symptoms of raised intracranial pressure (e.g. irritability, vomiting, headache, seizures and developmental delay) or exophthalmos.
- Neurosurgical intervention is indicated for raised intracranial pressure, progressive exophthalmos, or those at high risk of developing these complications. Cosmetic correction should only be contemplated for severe deformity.

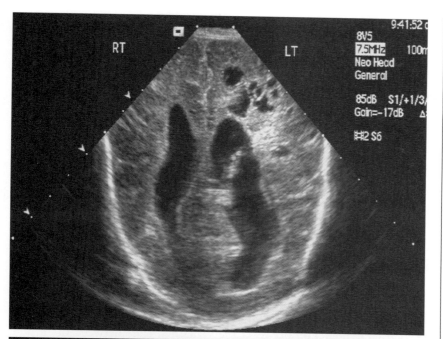

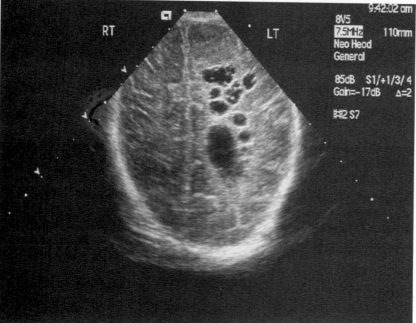

This baby was born at 28 weeks' gestation. This cranial ultrasound was performed at 4 weeks of age.

1. What does the ultrasound show?
2. What is the diagnosis?

ANSWERS

1. There are small cystic spaces in the left parietal lobe adjacent to the dilated left lateral ventricle. The surrounding parenchyma is of increased echogenicity.
2. Periventricular leucomalacia (PVL).

RADIOLOGY HOT LIST

- The earliest sign of PVL is increased periventricular echogenicity. However this can be a normal finding on neonatal cranial ultrasound, so the diagnosis may be missed if changes are subtle. Changes are often bilateral but asymmetrical.
- Cavitation occurs 1–6 weeks after the ischaemic insult, with small cystic spaces seen adjacent to the ventricles. There may be associated cerebral atrophy and ventriculomegaly.

CLINICAL HOT LIST

- Periventricular leucomalacia occurs after an ischaemic insult to the premature brain, which leads to tissue necrosis.
- Ischaemic infarction occurs at the watershed zone between the central and peripheral vascular supply.
- The prognosis is variable, ranging from mild intellectual impairment/ developmental delay to audiovisual deficit, epilepsy, cerebral palsy and microcephaly. Generalised PVL results in neurological deficit in nearly 100% of cases. Spastic diplegia or quadriplegia is more likely to be associated with this type of lesion.

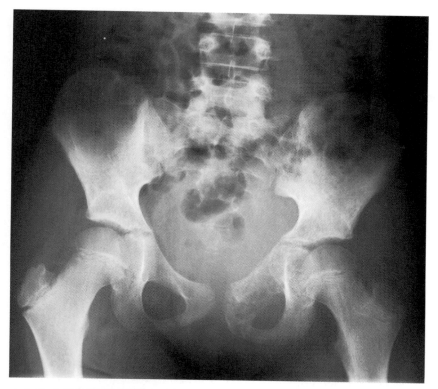

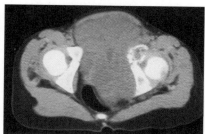
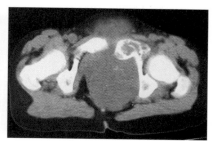

This 7 year old girl presented with left-sided limp and groin pain. An X-ray of the pelvis was requested, followed by a CT scan.

1. What does the plain film show?
2. What additional information is on the CT?
3. What is the diagnosis?

ANSWERS

1. The left superior pubic ramus is expanded, with an ill-defined and permeative abnormality of the bone texture. The left proximal femur is osteopenic, probably due to disuse osteoporosis.
2. There is an associated non-ossified soft tissue mass in the left hemipelvis, displacing the rectum to the right.
3. Ewing's sarcoma of the left superior pubic ramus.

RADIOLOGY HOT LIST

- Ewing's sarcoma occurs in the long bones in 60% (most commonly femur and tibia) and in the flat bones in 40% (pelvis and ribs).
- Plain films classically show a permeative, ill-defined lytic lesion with an associated soft tissue mass. There may be a periosteal reaction (classically lamellar 'onion-peel' but can also be spiculated 'sun-burst' pattern).
- MRI will assess the extent of marrow involvement and local extraosseous disease. Chest CT is required for the detection of pulmonary metastases, while a bone scan will detect skeletal metastases.
- Overlap occurs in the radiological appearances of Ewing's sarcoma and osteosarcoma. Infection and eosinophilic granuloma can occasionally give similar appearances on the plain film and a bone biopsy is required in all cases to establish histology.

CLINICAL HOT LIST

- Ewing's sarcoma is a malignant bone tumour of primitive small round cells. The peak incidence is 10–15 years.
- It presents with painful swelling at the affected site. Systemic symptoms may indicate metastatic disease.
- Features associated with a poor prognosis include metastases at diagnosis, proximal site (e.g. pelvis), soft tissue involvement and poor response to chemotherapy.
- Treatment: intensive chemotherapy followed by either surgery or radio-therapy.
- 8 year survival: 40% without metastases, 11% with metastases.

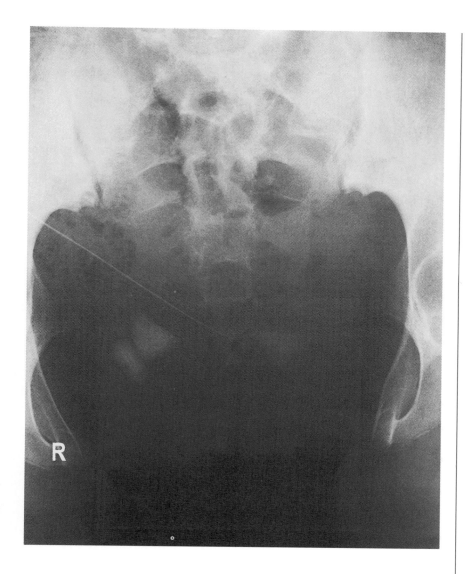

This 14 year old girl has been treated for multiple urinary tract infections since birth.

1. What does the X-ray of the pelvis show?
2. What is the diagnosis?

ANSWERS

1. The symphysis pubis is abnormally widened. There are three radio-opaque calculi present. There is also a suprapubic catheter in situ.
2. Bladder exstrophy, with bladder calculi present.

RADIOLOGY HOT LIST

- Gross widening of the symphysis pubis can be associated with a number of conditions including bladder exstrophy, epispadias and hypospadias, imperforate anus (with recto-vaginal fistula), urethral duplication and 'prune belly' syndrome.
- It is also a feature of some skeletal dysplasias.
- In bladder exstrophy bladder calculi form due to urinary stasis and infections.

CLINICAL HOT LIST

- Bladder exstrophy is a rare developmental disorder (1 : 40000) with incomplete mid-line closure of the infra-umbilical abdominal wall. It is often associated with other congenital abnormalities (limb, renal, GI, cardiac and neurological).
- The bladder is exposed and open anteriorly, with the mucosa everted through the defect in the anterior abdominal wall.
- It is associated with urinary incontinence, urinary tract infections and infertility.
- It is treated surgically with either a primary closure, or bladder excision and formation of a urinary diversion. Bilateral osteotomies may be required to bring the pubis together.

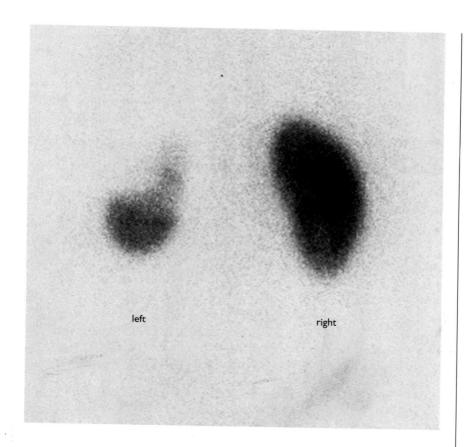

This study was obtained on a 10 year old girl under investigation for hypertension. An abdominal ultrasound had demonstrated a small non–obstructed left kidney but no other significant abnormality.

1. What is the examination?
2. What does it show?

ANSWERS

1. This is a technetium-99m DMSA scan.
2. The left kidney is small, with very poor tracer uptake (cold spots) in the upper pole and reduced uptake in the lower pole. The appearance is consistent with renal scarring. The right kidney appears normal.

RADIOLOGY HOT LIST

- DMSA is taken up in the proximal convoluted tubules, with minimal renal excretion. It accumulates in the renal cortex. Reduced uptake indicates areas of scarring (cortical loss). The relative amount of uptake by each kidney reflects differential function.
- DMSA scan is the investigation of choice for assessing renal scarring, which can be missed on an ultrasound investigation. (For further discussion see 'Rules and tools'.)

CLINICAL HOT LIST

- Blood pressure (BP) gradually increases through childhood, with most people following a constant percentile. Early childhood hypertension >95th percentile) usually has an underlying cause. Essential hypertension rarely occurs before adolescence (make sure an appropriate size paediatric BP cuff has been used!).
- Hypertension may be asymptomatic, or cause headaches, blurred vision, heart failure, stroke, seizures and coma.
- Causes of childhood hypertension:

Renal	dysplastic kidney, polycystic disease, obstructive uropathy, reflux nephropathy, glomerulonephritis, haemolytic-uraemic syndrome, Wilm's tumour
Endocrine	neuroblastoma, phaeochromocytoma, congenital adrenal hyperplasia, Cushing's syndrome, hyperaldosteronism
Vascular	aortic coarctation, renal artery stenosis, renal vein thrombosis, arteritis
Neurological	raised intracranial pressure, encephalitis

- Usual investigations include serum electrolyes and creatinine, urinanalysis, plasma and urine hormone/amine levels, and renal ultrasound.
- Treatment options are directed towards both the underlying cause and maintaining normal blood pressure. Hypertension can be controlled by a combination of diuretics, β-blockers and vasodilators. The prognosis depends on the underlying cause.

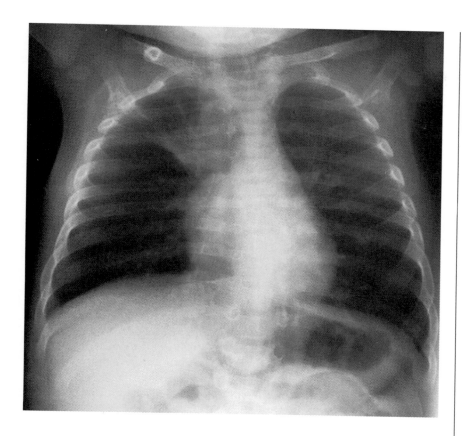

This 2 month old girl was seen in A&E with fever and wheeze. On examination she had tachypnoea, intercostal recession and widespread wheeze on auscultation.

1. What does the chest X-ray show?
2. What is the diagnosis?

ANSWERS

1. The lungs are hyperinflated. There is partial collapse of the right upper lobe (elevation of the horizontal fissure).
2. Bronchiolitis.

RADIOLOGY HOT LIST

- The chest X-ray in bronchiolitis may be normal. The commonest abnormality is hyperinflation (due to air trapping).
- There may be a 'dirty chest' appearance with peribronchial cuffing and interstitial infiltrates. Air space shadowing can also be seen, as well as any combination of lobar collapse and consolidation.
- Radiographic resolution may lag behind clinical resolution by 2–3 weeks.

CLINICAL HOT LIST

- It is the commonest lower respiratory tract infection in infancy. Peak incidence is at 3 months, and 2% require hospital admission.
- RSV is isolated in 75%, but there are many other potential viral pathogens.
- Clinical features include: coryza, low grade fever, cough, tachypnoea, wheeze, recession, hyperinflation and cyanosis. The disease is more severe in babies with an underlying cardiorespiratory disorder.
- Clinical differential diagnosis includes pneumonia, cardiac failure and aspiration.
- Treatment is supportive; oxygen therapy, witholding feeds, IV fluids and occasionally ventilation (1% of admissions). There is no clinically important benefit from steroids or bronchodilators.

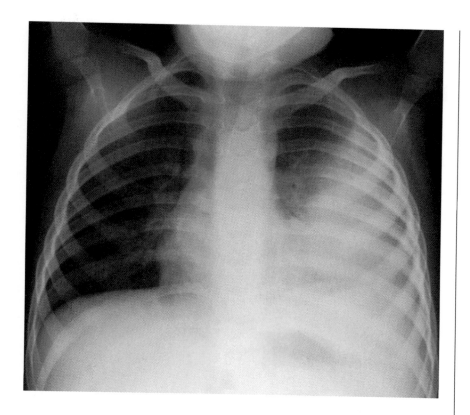

This 3 year old boy was treated by his GP for a chest infection for 1 week. He continued to be pyrexial, and a chest X-ray was obtained.

1. Name three abnormalities seen on the chest X-ray.
2. What is the diagnosis?

ANSWERS

1. In the left hemithorax there is dense opacification of the mid and lower zone, which has a curved superior margin. There is loss of the clarity of the left heart border and hemidiaphragm. The trachea is deviated to the right.
2. A large left pleural empyema, with left basal consolidation.

RADIOLOGY HOT LIST

● The appearance of pleural effusions in children may differ from that in adults – fluid often parallels the chest wall, appearing as a peripheral opaque band (lamellar effusion).

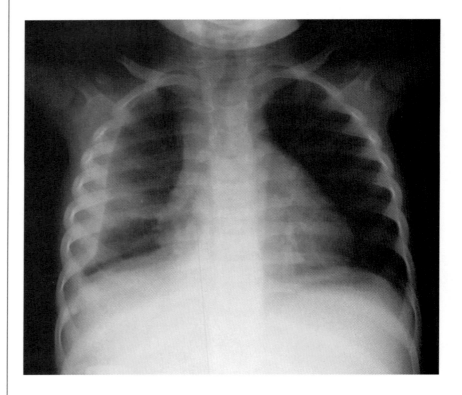

● Pleural effusions cause tracheal deviation **away** from the opaque hemi-thorax. There is often an associated pneumonic process in children, so look for areas of collapse and consolidation.
● Ultrasound will confirm the presence of fluid (anechoic in simple effusions), identify loculated collections, and guide percutaneous drainage.
● Contrast-enhanced CT scans will help to distinguish an empyema from a simple effusion by demonstrating enhancing pleural thickening in the former.

CLINICAL HOT LIST

- Simple reactive pleural effusions often complicate bacterial pneumonia. Superadded infection results in an empyema, which may require drainage (usually percutaneous, but surgical decortication may be required for complex organised collections).
- Causes of childhood pleural effusions:

Type of effusion	Causes
Transudate (protein <30 g/l)	cardiac failure, hepatic failure, nephrotic syndrome
Exudate (protein > 30 g/l)	infection, malignancy, infarction
Haemorrhagic	trauma, bleeding disorders

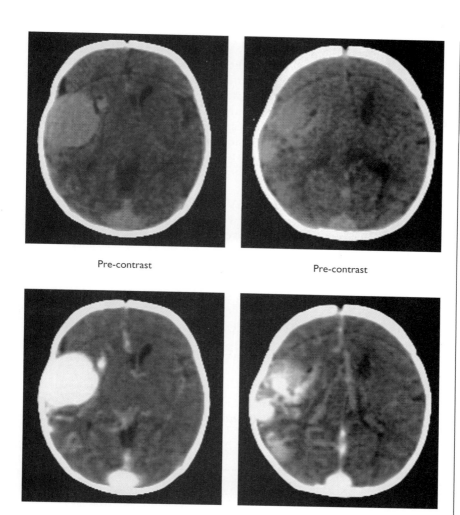

Pre-contrast

Pre-contrast

Post-contrast

Post-contrast

This 2 week old boy presented with high output cardiac failure.

1. What abnormalities are seen on the pre- and post-contrast CT scans of the brain?
2. What is the diagnosis?

ANSWERS

1. There is a round, well-circumscribed and hyperdense lesion in the right temporal lobe. It is causing mass effect with midline shift and effacement of the anterior horn of the right lateral ventricle. After contrast it shows intense uniform enhancement, with multiple adjacent abnormal vessels. The superior sagittal sinus shows early enhancement.
2. Right temporal arteriovenous malformation (AVM) with shunting.

RADIOLOGY HOT LIST

- Contrast-enhanced CT of an AVM will usually demonstrate dense enhancement, with large feeding vessels and draining veins. MRI will show characteristic areas of signal void in the vessels.
- A large AVM may cause obstructive hydrocephalus. Other complications include haemorrhage, infarction and local atrophy.
- A vein of Galen malformation is an AVM which arises in the midline and drains directly into an enlarged vein of Galen. It may be detected on antenatal ultrasound.
- Angiography may be necessary to define the vascular anatomy prior to surgery or embolisation.

CLINICAL HOT LIST

- AVMs are congenital abnormalities consisting of anomalous tortuous arteries and veins, creating an arteriovenous shunt without an intermediary capillary bed.
- Modes of presentation:

Age group	Typical presentation
Neonatal (0–1 month)	high output cardiac failure due to massive shunting
Infant (1–12 months)	obstructive hydrocephalus, seizures
>1 year	headaches, focal neurology, hydrocephalus, haemorrhage

- Therapeutic options include embolisation of arterial feeding vessels and complex neurosurgery.

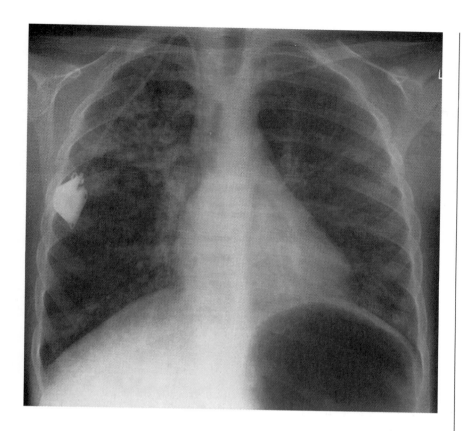

This child has been under long term follow-up for recurrent chest infections.

1. What abnormalities are seen on the chest radiograph?
2. What is the diagnosis?

ANSWERS

1. The lungs are hyperinflated, with widespread pulmonary infiltrates in all zones and bronchial wall thickening. There is ring shadowing due to bronchiectasis. There is a right-sided portacath in place.
2. Cystic fibrosis.

RADIOLOGY HOT LIST

- Typical features of cystic fibrosis on CXR include:

Bronchiectasis	parallel 'tram lines', ring shadows
Peribronchial thickening	thickened bronchial walls visible
Hyperinflation	low, flattened diaphragms
Mucus plugging	collapse, consolidation, air trapping
Fibrotic change	reticular–cystic pattern of fibrosis
Hilar lymphadenopathy and/or pulmonary artery dilatation secondary to pulmonary hypertension	prominent hila
Recurrent pneumonia	focal areas of collapse/consolidation
Long-term intravenous access	central venous lines, portacaths

- Be aware that in the early stages hyperinflation may be the only abnormality.
- Think of the diagnosis in a child with recurrent chest infections.

CLINICAL HOT LIST

- It is an autosomal recessive multisystem disorder, and the commonest cause of chronic lung disease and exocrine pancreatic insufficiency in childhood.
- Incidence (UK) is 1 : 2500, heterozygotes 1 : 25.
- It is due to a gene mutation on the long arm of chromsome 7, encoding for the cystic fibrosis transmembrane conductance regulator. >450 gene mutations identified, 70% ΔF508.
- Presentations include chronic respiratory symptoms, recurrent chest infections, failure to thrive, meconium ileus, malabsorption with steatorrhea, rectal prolapse and nasal polyps.
- Management strategies include diet, pancreatic supplements, physiotherapy, appropriate antibiotics, bronchodilators and DNAase.
- Survival is 75% to 18 years with good care.

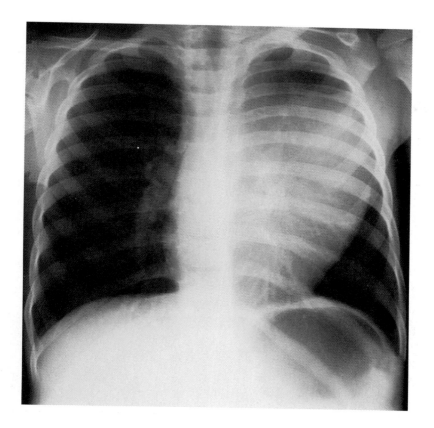

This two and a half year old boy presented to his GP with a 4 week history of lethargy, fever and night sweats.

1. What abnormality is seen on the chest X-ray?
2. What is the most likely diagnosis?
3. What is the differential diagnosis?

ANSWERS

1. There is a soft tissue mass projected over the left hemithorax. The left heart border and superior mediastial outlines are obscured, but the hilum is visible through the mass. This indicates that the mass lies in the anterior mediastinum.
2. Lymphoma.
3. Leukaemia, inflammatory lymphadenopathy (secondary to tuberculosis), germ cell tumours and thymic masses.

RADIOLOGY HOT LIST

- Mediastinal masses have a wide differential, and it is useful to consider them according to their anatomical location – superior, anterior, middle, or posterior mediastinum. This can often be determined on the plain X-ray, but most children will proceed to CT scan for further assessment.
- Hodgkin's disease accounts for the majority of neoplastic anterior mediastinal masses in children. TB is a common non-neoplastic cause of mediastinal node enlargement.

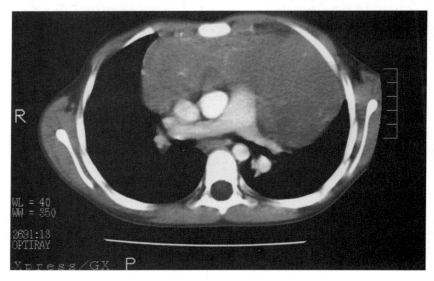

CT scan showing an anterior mediastinal mass due to lymphoma.

CLINICAL HOT LIST

- At the time of presentation, mediastinal lymph nodes are seen in 25% of children with Hodgkin's lymphoma, 15% with non-Hodgkin's lymphoma, and 5–10% with leukaemia. A residual mass (which may demonstrate eggshell calcification post-radiotherapy) may persist after treatment and should be followed up.
- Lung involvement is present in 10% of Hodgkin's disease, but is more common in non-Hodgkin's lymphoma (disseminated at presentation in 75%).

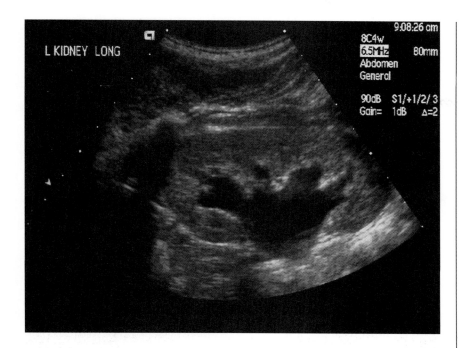

This renal ultrasound was performed on a 2 day old baby girl for an antenatally detected condition.

1. What abnormality is seen in the left kidney?
2. What is the diagnosis?

ANSWERS

1. There is dilatation of the left pelvicalyceal system (black anechoic areas).
2. Hydronephrosis.

RADIOLOGY HOT LIST

- The calyces are only seen on ultrasound when distended by fluid.
- Ultrasound cannot reliably distinguish between the two most important causes of hydronephrosis: obstruction and vesicoureteric reflux. Further imaging studies (micturating cystourethrogram and/or nuclear medicine studies) are required to differentiate the conditions.
- If antenatal hydronephrosis is detected, postnatal follow-up is mandatory, in order to exclude reflux (up to 30%), and other urological abnormalities such as posterior urethral valves and pelvi-ureteric junction obstruction. Local practice varies.
- A normal postnatal ultrasound does not exclude reflux.

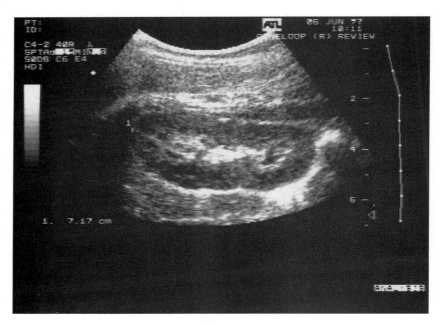

Ultrasound appearance of a normal kidney.

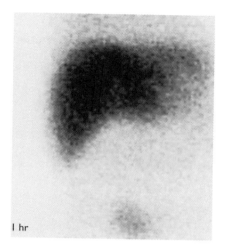
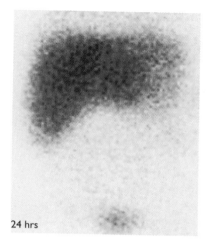

1 hr

24 hrs

This 3 week old boy was noted by the community midwife to have prolonged jaundice. Ultrasound showed a non-dilated biliary tree but the gallbladder was not visualised. This HIDA scan (hepatic nuclear medicine scan) was carried out as part of his investigations.

1. What does it show?
2. What is the diagnosis?
3. What is the differential diagnosis for this presentation?

ANSWERS

1. The HIDA scan shows uptake of tracer by the liver, but no excretion into the small bowel. The appearance remains unchanged over 24 hours. (Normal activity is seen in the urinary bladder.)

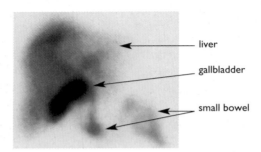

Normal HIDA scan, showing activity in the gallbladder and small bowel at 20 minutes.

2. Biliary atresia.
3. Other causes for persistent neonatal jaundice include 'breast milk' jaundice, hepatitis and choledocal cyst.

RADIOLOGY HOT LIST

- Ultrasound examination is the initial radiological investigation for persisting jaundice, in order to differentiate between obstructive and non-obstructive causes.
- The presence of a gallbladder makes biliary atresia much less likely (gall-bladder only present in 20%). The biliary tree is typically not dilated in biliary atresia.
- A choledocal cyst is usually suspected from the ultrasound appearances.
- MR cholangiopancreatography may demonstrate the intra- and extra-hepatic biliary tree.
- Polysplenia is associated with biliary atresia (10%).

CLINICAL HOT LIST

- Causes of persisting jaundice include – breast feeding (up to 6 weeks), hepatitis (due to infections such as toxoplasmosis, rubella and cyto-megalovirus), choledocal cyst, metabolic abnormalities and inborn errors of metabolism.
- Biliary atresia occurs more commonly in male infants (2 : 1).
- Liver biopsy may be necessary to distinguish between biliary atresia and neonatal hepatitis.
- Cirrhosis develops if untreated within 60 days. Early surgery (Kasai procedure – portoenterostomy) is the definitive treatment. Where this is not possible (or too late), transplantation is the only alternative.

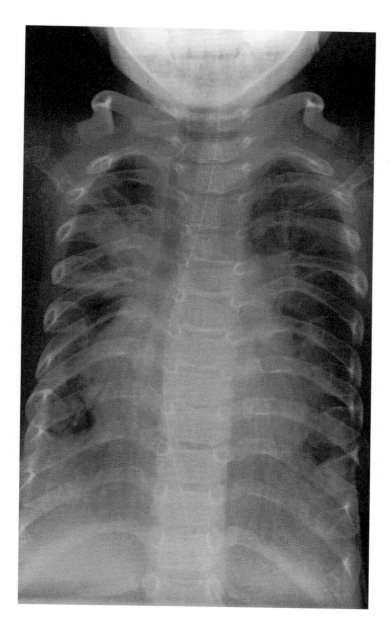

This baby girl presented with respiratory difficulties in the neonatal period, which have persisted. The midwife had noted that her limbs were short, but there were no other dysmorphic features.

1. Comment on the CXR.
2. What is the most likely diagnosis?
3. What is the prognosis?

ANSWERS

1. The thoracic cage is narrow with small volume lungs. The ribs are short and horizontal with broad and expanded anterior ends. There is consolidation in the right upper lobe.
2. Jeune's thoracic dystrophy.
3. Generally poor prognosis – most die from respiratory failure before 1 year of age.

RADIOLOGY HOT LIST

- Classically elongated and bell-shaped chest with normal heart size, leaving little room for the lungs.
- Short horizontal ribs and irregular bulbous costochondral junctions.
- Other skeletal abnormalities: 'wineglass' pelvis with short flared iliac bones and reduced acetabular angle, rhizomelia, postaxial hexadactyly, short phalanges and metaphyseal irregularity.
- Look for features of respiratory tract infection.

CLINICAL HOT LIST

- It is autosomal recessive chondrodysplasia, predominantly affecting the costochondral junctions.
- The differential diagnosis for a small thorax with other skeletal abnormalities includes thanatophoric dwarfism and Ellis van Creveld syndrome.

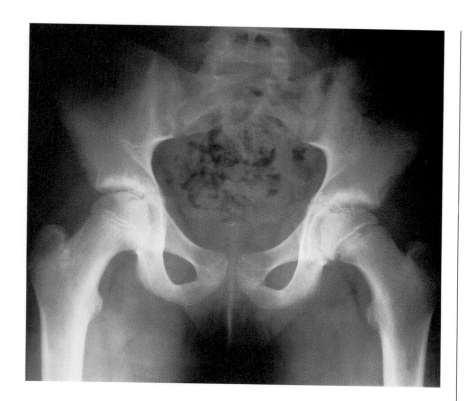

This 14 year old girl presented to A&E with a 2 week history of left-sided limp.

1. What is the diagnosis?

ANSWERS

1. There is a slipped femoral capital epiphysis on the left.

RADIOLOGY HOT LIST

- Epiphyseal slip may be difficult to identify on the plain AP X-ray. It is usually more obvious on the frog lateral view, which should be obtained in older children with hip pain.
- The slip is posteromedial in 99% of cases.
- Radiographic signs:
  —widening of the epiphyseal plate.
  —reduction in the apparent height of the epiphysis.
  —a line drawn tangential to the lateral border of the femoral neck should normally pass through the lateral aspect of the femoral capital epiphysis.
  —displacement of the medial femoral metaphysis so that it no longer overlies the acetabulum.

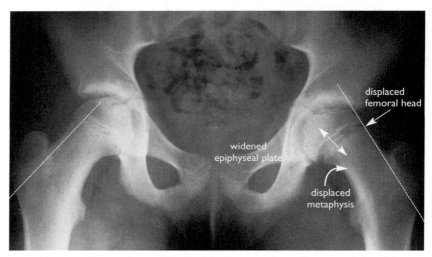

Normal hip on right and abnormal hip on left showing radiographic signs of slipped femoral epiphysis.

CLINICAL HOT LIST

- It classically occurs at the time of the pubertal growth spurt (girls age 10–13 years, boys age 12–15 years). There is an increased incidence in boys and overweight children. Bilateral slip is present in 20–40% cases.
- Treatment aims to prevent further slippage rather than repositioning the slipped femoral head. There must be limitation of activity but prophylactic surgical pinning may be required. The pins are usually removed after growth plate fusion.
- Complications include avascular necrosis, acute cartilage necrosis, premature physeal closure with subsequent limb–length discrepancy, and premature osteoarthritis.

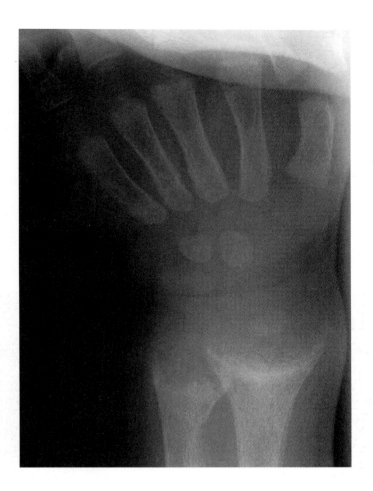

This 18 month old baby has swollen wrists.

1. What does the X-ray show?
2. What is the diagnosis?

ANSWERS

1. There is cupping, fraying and irregularity of the metaphyses of the distal radius and ulna.
2. Rickets.

RADIOLOGY HOT LIST

- Radiological change is seen at the distal ends of long bones, at the sites of most rapid growth: changes are most evident at the wrists and knees. There may be cupping of the anterior ribs at the costochondral junction ('rickety rosary').
- Look for leg bowing in weight-bearing children, pathological fractures, generalised osteopenia and skull bossing in severe cases.
- The radiological manifestations of rickets cannot reliably distinguish between the different aetiologies.
- Rickets may be an incidental finding on the chest X-ray – always look at the humeral metaphyses.

CLINICAL HOT LIST

- Failure of mineralisation of osteoid leads to bone softening and deformity.
- Classification of rickets:

Nutritional	dietary deficiency of vitamin D or lack of sunlight
Malabsorption	coeliac disease, hepatobiliary disease
Hereditary renal	X-linked hypophosphataemia, vitamin D-dependent rickets, Fanconi's syndrome, distal renal tubular acidosis
Acquired renal	chronic renal failure
Neonatal rickets (rare)	prematurity, copper deficiency, secondary to maternal osteomalacia

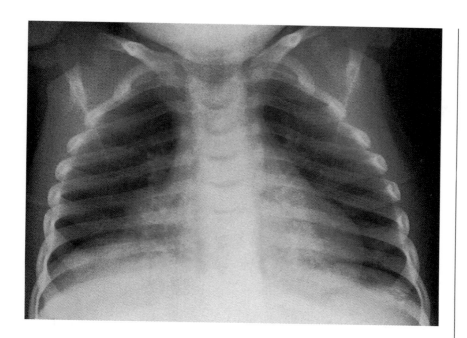

This 2 year old boy has a cough and fever.

1. What does the chest X-ray show?
2. What is the diagnosis?

ANSWERS

1. There is consolidation in the right mid zone which obscures the right heart border. The rest of the lungs are clear.
2. Right middle lobe pneumonia.

RADIOLOGY HOT LIST

- The heart borders and diaphragm are clear and distinct on a chest X-ray as they are interfaces between radiolucent air (lung) and radio-opaque soft tissue.
- Opacification of the lung secondary to consolidation or collapse results in loss of the air–soft tissue interface – hence the ill-defined margins. The site of lung pathology can be predicted by which interface is obliterated.

Obscured interface	Lung lobe involved
Right heart border	Right middle lobe
Right hemidiaphragm	Right lower lobe
Right paratracheal	Right upper lobe
Left heart border	Lingula (left upper lobe)
Left hemidiaphragm	Left lower lobe

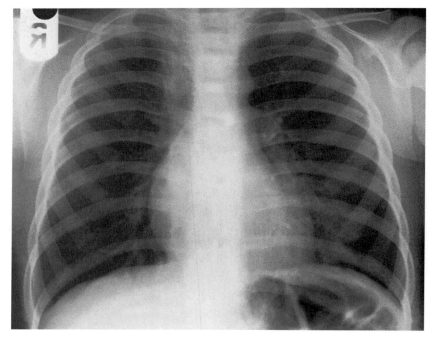

Right upper lobe collapse with widening of the right superior mediastinum, and loss of the well-defined right paratracheal stripe.

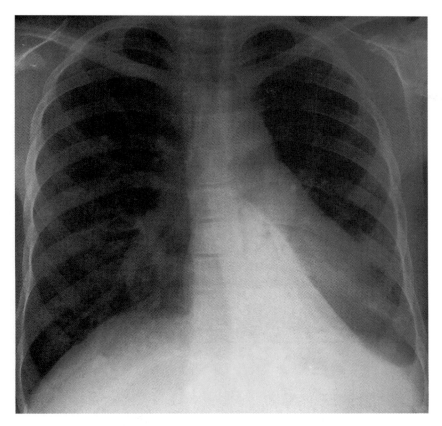

Left lower lobe collapse causing a triangular-shaped density behind the heart, and loss of the normal medial left hemidiaphragm contour.

- Children may also develop round pneumonias – rounded focal areas of consolidation, which have the appearance of a mass lesion. Follow up chest X-rays show resolution after antibiotic therapy.

CLINICAL HOT LIST

- Lobar consolidation is usually due to bacterial infection, with *pneumococcus* most commonly implicated. *Haemophilus*, *mycoplasma* and primary tuberculosis can give a similar appearance. *Klebsiella* infection classically shows 'bulging' of adjacent fissures.

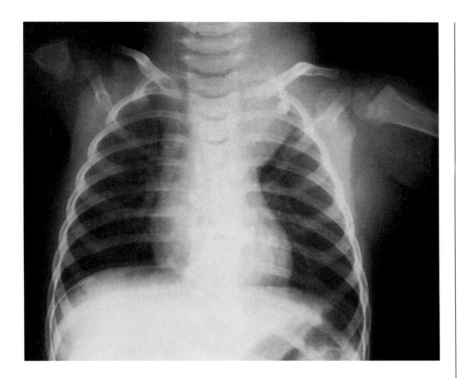

This 18 month old girl with Turner's syndrome has a neck swelling extending into the axilla.

1. What does the chest X-ray show?
2. What is the most likely diagnosis?

ANSWERS

1. There is a large well-circumscribed soft tissue mass on the left side of the neck, extending into the axilla and into the superior mediastinum. It displaces the trachea to the right.
2. Cystic hygroma.

RADIOLOGY HOT LIST

- The mass extends from the neck into the superior mediastinum and displaces the trachea – this distinguishes it from a normal thymus gland, which does not extend above the thoracic inlet and causes no tracheal deviation.

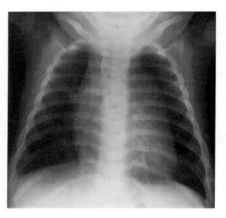

Chest X-ray showing a normal thymus.

- A cystic hygroma appears as a thin-walled fluid structure on ultrasound. Internal septations may be present.
- MRI shows a T2-weighted high signal, and may show a fluid–fluid level if there has been previous haemorrhage.

CLINICAL HOT LIST

- Cystic hygromas are single or multiloculated fluid-filled structures. They arise in the neck, and may extend into the thorax or involve the trunk. They are caused by a congenital blockage of lymphatic drainage. 50% present at birth, most by 2 years.
- Associations: Turner's syndrome (40–80%), trisomies (13,18,21), Noonan's syndrome, previous exposure to teratogens (e.g. fetal alcohol syndrome).
- There may be compression of the airway and/or oesophagus. Sudden enlargement may occur due to haemorrhage or infection.
- There is a high incidence of fetal demise (33%). Spontaneous regression occurs in 15%. Localised lesions are associated with a favourable prognosis. Surgical excision is technically difficult.

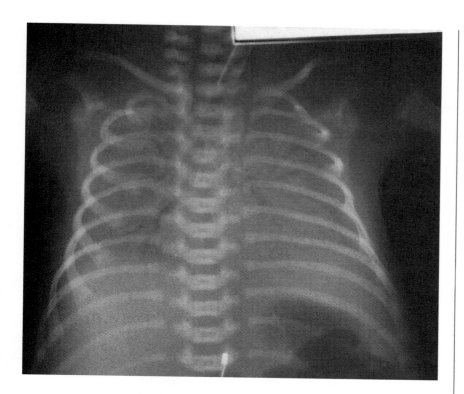

This baby was born at 26 weeks' gestation, and ventilated for respiratory distress. This chest X-ray was taken at 36 hours.

1. What abnormalities are seen?
2. What is the most likely diagnosis?
3. What is the differential diagnosis?

ANSWERS

1. The lungs are small volume. There is diffuse symmetrical granular opacification of both lungs ('ground glass'), with bilateral air bronchograms, and loss of clarity of the cardiac outline and diaphragm. There is an endotracheal tube in situ.
2. Hyaline membrane disease (HMD).
3. Neonatal pneumonia, pulmonary haemorrhage.

RADIOLOGY HOT LIST

- The chest X-ray in HMD may be normal initially, but is usually abnormal by 6 hours.
- The chest X-ray may progress from fine reticular shadowing to complete white-out with air bronchograms and loss of the cardiac and diaphragmatic contours.
- Radiological findings are usually symmetrical, but this may not be true following ventilation or surfactant therapy.

CLINICAL HOT LIST

- HMD refers to the histological appearance and is synonymous with respiratory distress syndrome. Lack of surfactant causes diffuse alveolar collapse.
- It is common under 30 weeks gestation and almost inevitable under 28 weeks.
- Other associations include asphyxia, hypothermia, haemolytic disease of the newborn and maternal diabetes.
- The incidence can be reduced by prevention of premature delivery and antenatal maternal steroids.
- Neonatal pneumonia may have an indistinguishable appearance from HMD, and antibiotic cover is required until the results of blood cultures are known.

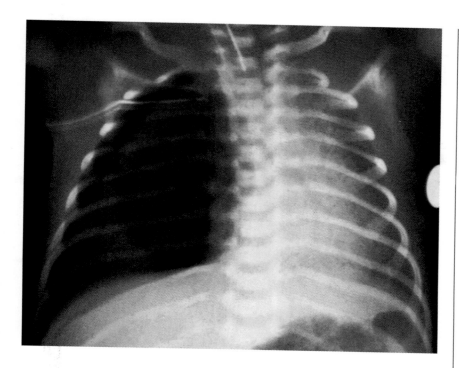

This 5 day old baby, born at 28 weeks' gestation and ventilated for hyaline membrane disease (HMD), had a sudden onset of increasing oxygen and ventilatory requirements.

1. What abnormality is seen on the chest radiograph?
2. What is the diagnosis?

ANSWERS

1. There is a right-sided pneumothorax with mediastinal shift and depression of the diaphragm. The underlying lung is stiff (due to HMD) and has not collapsed. The large lucency projected over the lung is the anterior component of the pneumothorax. A right intercostal drain and an endotracheal tube are in situ.
2. Neonatal pneumothorax complicating hyaline membrane disease.

RADIOLOGY HOT LIST

- Neonatal pneumothorax may not have the classic appearances seen in ambulant children because the film is taken with the baby supine.
- The lung is usually displaced posteriorly in the supine patient, with free pleural air collecting anteriorly and medially. Thus the AP film may only show increased radiolucency over the entire hemithorax, or a sharp outline to the adjacent mediastinum. A lung edge may not be seen.
- There may be a subpulmonary collection of air.
- Look for mediastinal shift, pneumomediastinum and subcutaneous emphysema.
- If the underlying lung is stiff (e.g. from HMD) it may not collapse completely.

CLINICAL HOT LIST

- Spontaneous pneumothorax is most common in the neonatal period. Many will go undetected as they are clinically silent. The incidence of iatrogenic pneumothorax in ventilated babies is decreasing as a result of surfactant and improved ventilator strategies.
- Associations include mechanical ventilation, HMD, pulmonary interstitial emphysema and meconium aspiration.
- Management depends on clinical severity; the vast majority of ventilated neonates will require a chest drain.

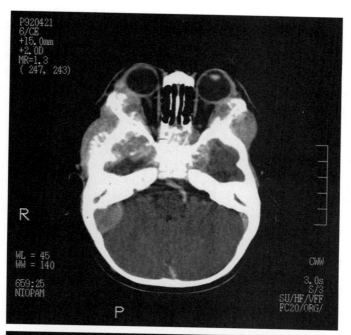

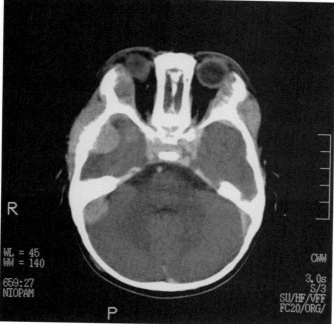

This 1 year old boy presented with proptosis, hypertension and an abdominal mass.

1. What does the contrast–enhanced CT scan show?
2. What is the most likely diagnosis?

ANSWERS

1. There are enhancing, extracerebral masses in the middle and posterior cranial fossae. There is new bone formation with a spiculated periosteal reaction in the skull base and both lateral orbital walls. There is abnormal retro-orbital and extracranial soft tissue. There is bilateral proptosis.
2. Metastatic bony, orbital and parameningeal neuroblastoma deposits.

RADIOLOGY HOT LIST

- Bone metastases are common in children over 1 year of age with neuroblastoma. They mainly involve the long bones and orbits (classically the lateral wall).
- Parameningeal deposits are less common, and are secondary to haematogenous spread to the epidural space.
- Rhabdomyosarcoma may also affect the orbit, but is usually unilateral and there may be extensive bone destruction.

CLINICAL HOT LIST

- Neuroblastoma is the most common extracranial solid malignant tumour in children.
- Neuroblastoma may remain clinically silent until it causes mass effect, invades neighbouring structures, or metastasizes.
- 70% of patients have disseminated disease at diagnosis, and many presenting symptoms are secondary to metastatic spread. Proptosis and bone pain are well-recognised clinical presentations.

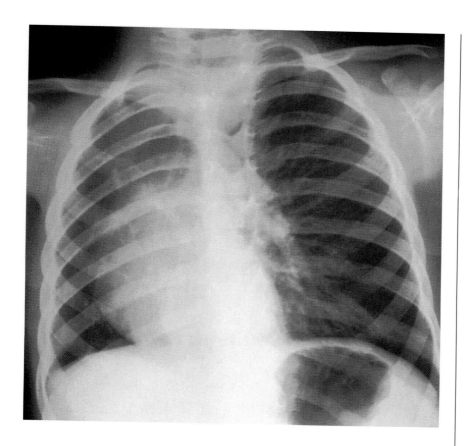

This 4 year old boy is asymptomatic.

1. What does the chest X-ray show?
2. What is the diagnosis?

ANSWERS

1. The right hemithorax is reduced in volume and there is mediastinal shift to this side. The right lung has reduced vascularity (right main pulmonary artery not seen and paucity of vessels peripherally). No focal areas of collapse or consolidation.
2. Right pulmonary hypoplasia.

RADIOLOGY HOT LIST

- Common causes of mediastinal shift

| Towards affected side | collapse secondary to an inhaled foreign body, mucous plug or infection. Pulmonary hypoplasia |
| Away from affected side | air trapping due to an inhaled foreign body, tension pneumothorax, large pleural effusion, intrathoracic mass |

- Always assess the pulmonary vasculature. The oligaemic side is usually the abnormal side!
- The small hemithorax and mediastinal shift, coupled with the diminished vascularity, indicate chronic pathology, rather than an acute pulmonary collapse. Always compare with old films.
- Distinguish this from McCloud's syndrome with a small pulmonary artery, oligaemia, **but** air trapping and a large/normal volume hemithorax.

CLINICAL HOT LIST

- Congenital underdevelopment of one or more lobes of the lung can be differentiated into three forms:

Pulmonary agenesis	absence of lobe and bronchus
Pulmonary aplasia	rudimentary bronchus with no parenchyma or vessels
Pulmonary hypoplasia	bronchus completely formed, but small. Small vessels and rudimentary parenchyma

- Idiopathic pulmonary hypoplasia is often asymptomatic and an incidental finding on chest X-rays. Patients may be prone to exertional dyspnoea.

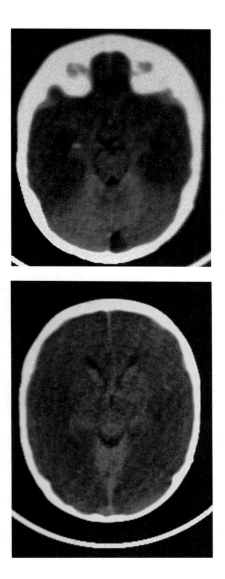

This term infant was born after emergency Caesarean section for a placental abruption. At delivery, he was white, floppy and had a profound brady-cardia. He was resuscitated, but has had frequent seizures since his admission to the neonatal unit. This scan was taken 48 hours after birth.

1. What does the CT brain scan show?
2. What is the diagnosis?

ANSWERS

1. There is diffuse low density in both cerebral hemispheres with loss of the normal grey-white matter differentiation (due to global cerebral oedema). The cerebellum, basal ganglia and thalamus appear relatively high density – the 'acute reversal sign'.
2. Hypoxic–ischaemic encephalopathy.

RADIOLOGY HOT LIST

- Severe hypoxic–ischaemic encephalopathy may manifest as the 'acute reversal sign' on CT. This occurs due to relative preservation of cerebral perfusion to the brainstem, cerebellum and basal ganglia after the hypoxic insult.
- These features may occur after any cause of hypoxic–ischaemic insult, including non–accidental injury.
- The acute reversal sign on CT indicates a poor prognosis: survivors usually have severe neurological deficit.
- MRI may be of value in the assessment of these patients.

CLINICAL HOT LIST

- Causes of hypoxic ischaemic encephalopathy:

Medical causes	birth asphyxia, meningitis, encephalitis, status epilepticus, status asthmaticus, drowning, cardiac arrest
Trauma	accidental or non-accidental (shaking/smothering injuries)

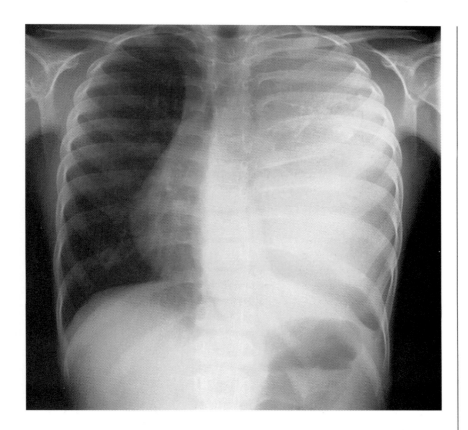

This 5 year old girl has become increasingly short of breath and tired.

1. What does the chest X-ray show?
2. What is the diagnosis?

ANSWERS

1. The left hemithorax is radiopaque and small areas of calcification are seen within it. There is loss of the left heart border and mediastinal shift to the right. The posterior ribs are splayed and eroded, indicating the presence of an aggressive mass lesion.
2. Thoracic neuroblastoma.

RADIOLOGY HOT LIST

- Neurogenic tumours account for 95% of posterior mediastinal masses in children.
- Look for calcification (25% of thoracic neuroblastomas) and associated vertebral or rib erosion.
- MRI or CT is required to assess anatomical location and spread.

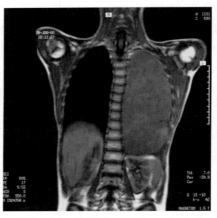

Coronal T1-weighted MRI through the patient's thorax.

- Look for extension into the spinal canal (extradural extension).
- Other causes of posterior mediastinal masses in children include paraspinal abscess, extramedullary haematopoeisis, oeophageal duplication cyst, or a neuroenteric cyst (associated with vertebral anomalies).

CLINICAL HOT LIST

- 15% of neuroblastomas occur in the thorax, arising from the sympathetic ganglia.
- Neuroblastoma is often clinically silent until it invades or compresses adjacent structures, such as the trachea or oesophagus.
- Extradural spread may cause spinal cord compression with paraplegia, Horner's syndrome, or alteration in bladder or bowel function. The tumour may require irradiation and chemotherapy prior to surgical excision.
- Thoracic neuroblastoma has a significantly better prognosis, probably due to earlier clinical presentation.

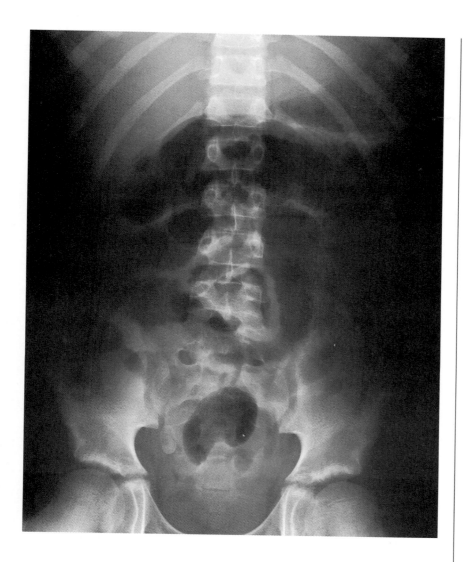

This 12 year old boy was admitted via A&E with fever, abdominal pain and vomiting.

1. Identify two abnormalities present on the plain abdominal X-ray.
2. What is the diagnosis?

ANSWERS

1. There are centrally located and distended bowel loops, consistent with an ileus. There is an opacity projected over the right lower quadrant, typical of an appendicolith.
2. Acute appendicitis.

RADIOLOGY HOT LIST

- The plain abdominal X-ray may be normal in >50%, but the presence of an appendicolith in a child with abdominal pain gives >90% probability of appendicitis.
- There may be small bowel dilatation secondary to an ileus.
- An appendix abscess may be detected as a soft tissue mass, or a paucity of bowel loops in the right iliac fossa, and may be associated with extra-luminal gas.
- Ultrasound may be diagnostic and may demonstrate any of the following: a typical tubular structure with a cross-section diameter >6 mm, a complex mass, appendicolith, free fluid.
- The diagnosis is not excluded by negative imaging.

CLINICAL HOT LIST

- It is the commonest surgical emergency of childhood.
- Symptoms in older children are similar to those seen in adults. The cardinal sign is tenderness at McBurney's point. However, in younger children presentation may be with anorexia, fever, diarrhoea and vomiting.
- The differential diagnosis includes non-specific abdominal pain, gastro-enteritis, mesenteric adenitis, Henoch–Schönlein purpura, constipation, urinary tract infection, lower lobe pneumonia and diabetes.
- Treatment consists of resuscitation and appendicectomy. An appendix mass may be managed conservatively.

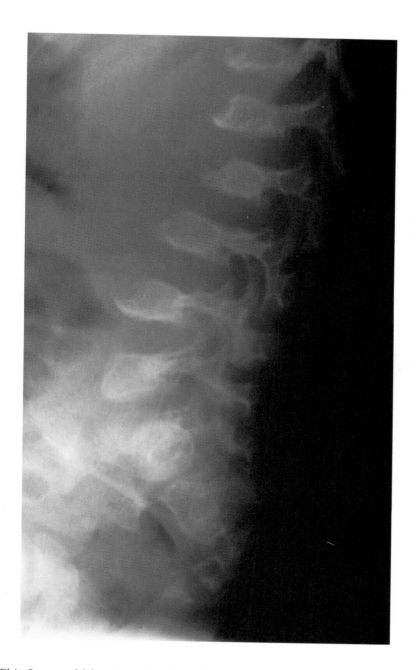

This 2 year old boy is under investigation for progressive developmental retardation. On examination he is short, has coarse facial features and hepatosplenomegaly.

1. What does the lateral X-ray of the lumbar spine show?
2. What is the most likely diagnosis?
3. What is the differential diagnosis?

ANSWERS

1. There is a mild kyphosis at the thoracolumbar junction. The vertebral bodies are abnormal with anterior inferior beaking and long slender pedicles.
2. Mucopolysaccharidosis: Hurler's syndrome.
3. Other causes of anterior inferior beaking of the vertebral bodies include achondroplasia and hypothyroidism.

RADIOLOGY HOT LIST

- Skeletal dysplasia is a component of Hurler's syndrome, with widespread radiographic abnormalities involving the axial skeleton and the extremities.
- The earliest radiographic changes involve the skull: frontal bossing, calvarial thickening and a J-shaped sella. The characteristic features in the spine are described above. The iliac bones are flared. The ribs are 'oar shaped'.
- The hands are abnormal ('trident hands'): broad expanded metacarpals with tapered proximal ends.

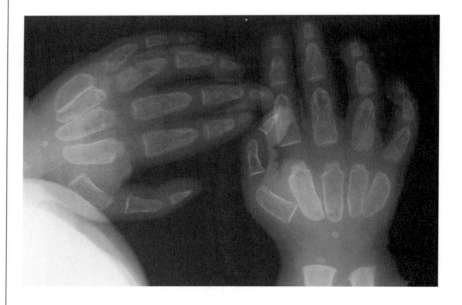

CLINICAL HOT LIST

- The mucopolysaccharidoses are a complex heterogeneous group of lysosomal storage disorders, with abnormalities of mucopolysaccharide or glycoprotein metabolism.
- Classification depends on the particular enzyme deficiency. There are seven types in total. Babies are usually normal at birth, but develop multisystem disease by 2 years.

Type	Inheritance	Neurological signs	Somatic features	Prognosis
I–Hurler	Autosomal recessive	Marked retardation	Coarse facies, short stature, skeletal dysplasia, corneal clouding, hepatosplenomegaly, valvular heart disease	Death in childhood, bone marrow transplantation curative
II–Hunter	X-linked	Mild retardation	As for Hurler's (but no corneal clouding)	Survive to adulthood
IV–Morquio	Autosomal dominant	Normal	Normal face, short stature, marked kyphosis, hypotonia, contractures	Survive to adulthood

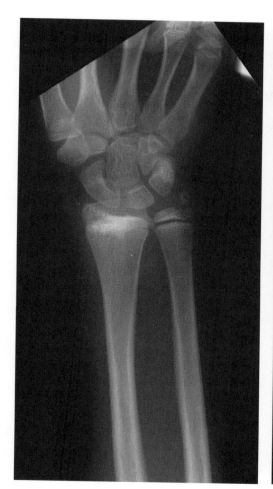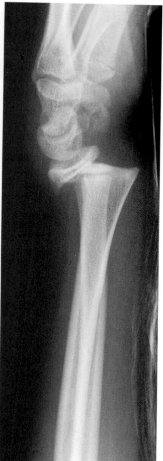

A 13 year old boy was brought to casualty following an injury on the football pitch.

1. What abnormality is demonstrated on the plain radiograph?
2. What is the diagnosis?
3. What is the significance of recognising this injury?

ANSWERS

1. There is posterior displacement of the distal radial epiphysis, which is only appreciated on the lateral view. This illustrates the importance of two views at right angles when assessing trauma.
2. A Salter Harris type I epiphyseal injury.
3. Epiphyseal fractures may require open reduction to avoid angulation and/or premature fusion with consequent limb shortening.

RADIOLOGY HOT LIST

- The epiphyseal complex (epiphysis, cartilagenous growth plate, and metaphysis) is involved in 6–15% of paediatric fractures, most commonly at the wrist and the ankle.
- It is important to recognise fractures involving the growth plate as orthopaedic intervention may be required.

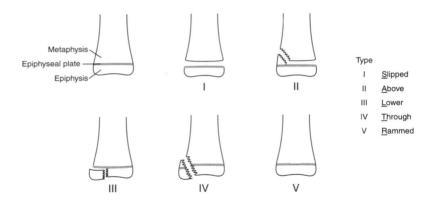

Type	
I	Slipped
II	Above
III	Lower
IV	Through
V	Rammed

SALTR – This is a useful mnemonic, describing the relation of the fracture to the epiphyseal plate.

CLINICAL HOT LIST

- Types I, II and III fractures are treated by closed reduction and immobilisation.
- Types IV and V fractures require open reduction and internal fixation to prevent premature growth plate fusion with subsequent limb shortening and angulation.

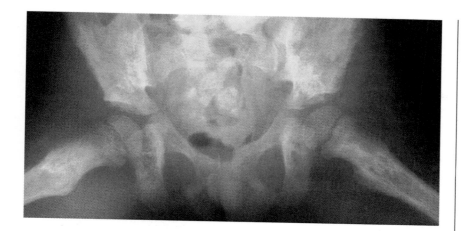

This 5 year old boy presented with right-sided hip pain and bruising. The full blood count showed anaemia and thrombocytopaenia, but a high white cell count.

1. Comment on the X-ray of the pelvis.
2. What is the diagnosis?

ANSWERS

1. The bone texture is diffusely abnormal throughout, with a permeative, moth-eaten appearance. There are bilateral symmetrical periosteal reactions along both femoral shafts.
2. Acute lymphoblastic leukaemia.

RADIOLOGY HOT LIST

- Skeletal manifestations occur in 50–90% of leukaemia patients and are usually due to leukaemic infiltration. X-ray changes may precede blood film abnormalities, and resolve with successful therapy.
- The appearances may include osteoporosis, transverse lucent metaphyseal bands, focal osteolytic lesions and periosteal reactions.
- Similar radiological features are seen with metastatic neuroblastoma.

CLINICAL HOT LIST

Pathology	Clinical manifestation
Bone marrow failure	Anaemia, thrombocytopaenia, neutropenia
Tissue and organ infiltration	Splenomegaly, lymphadenopathy, bone involvement
Systemic effects	Fever, lethargy, anorexia

- Treatment includes chemotherapy, radiotherapy, bone marrow transplantation and supportive measures (blood transfusions and prevention/treatment of infection).

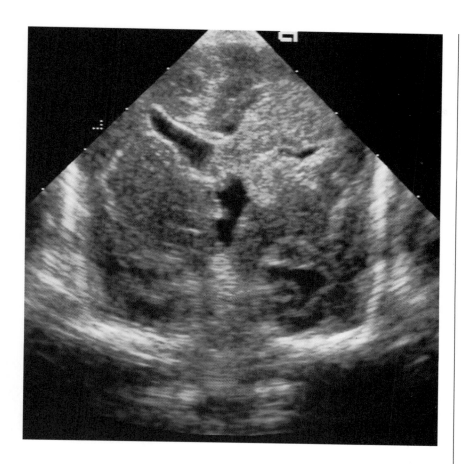

This 3 day old baby was born at 27 weeks' gestation and ventilated for severe hyaline membrane disease. He suddenly collapsed on the ventilator with hypotension, metabolic acidosis and hypotonia. A cranial ultrasound scan was performed.

1. What abnormality is seen?
2. What are the possible sequelae to this?

ANSWERS

1. There is a mass of increased echogenicity seen in the left lateral ventricle with extension into the left frontal lobe. This represents a grade IV intraventricular haemorrhage with parenchymal extension. There is dilatation of the left temporal horn secondary to the obstructing clot.
2. Large haemorrhages may cause hydrocephalus, encephalomalacia, neurological impairment and death.

RADIOLOGY HOT LIST

- The echogenic choroid plexus does not extend beyond the caudothalamic groove, so any high echogenicity seen in the anterior horns of the lateral ventricles is pathological.
- The blood clot appears as an amorphous mass of high echogenicity which may fill the ventricle, or layer in the dependent part of the ventricle.
- Assess ventricular dilatation, and the adjoining cerebral parenchyma for periventricular involvement.
- Classification:

Grade 1	Confined to subependymal germinal matrix
Grade 2	Extension into non-dilated ventricles
Grade 3	Extension into dilated ventricles
Grade 4	Massive intraventricular and intraparenchymal haemorrhage

CLINICAL HOT LIST

- Haemorrhage occurs in the germinal layer (vascular network, floor of lateral ventricles). This normally involutes in the later part of pregnancy, and thus periventricular haemorrhage (PVH) is not usually seen in infants over 32 weeks gestation.
- It affects 20% of neonates with a birth weight below 1.5 kg.
- It is commonly asymptomatic, particularly grade 1 and 2, and therefore routine scanning is necessary on neonatal intensive care units.
- Risk factors include hypotension, hypoxia, acidosis, respiratory distress syndrome and pneumothorax.
- Grades 1 and 2 have a good prognosis. Virtually all those with grade 4 lesions will have neurological impairment.

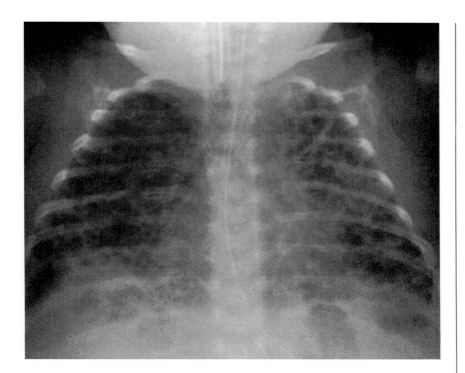

This 5 week old baby was born at 26 weeks' gestation and has been ventilated since birth.

1. What abnormalities are seen on the chest X-ray?
2. What is the diagnosis?

ANSWERS

1. The lungs are hyperinflated. There is coarse reticular shadowing with rounded lucent areas in both lungs. The heart and diaphragmatic outlines are ill defined.
2. Bronchopulmonary dysplasia.

RADIOLOGY HOT LIST

- Bronchopulmonary dysplasia is defined as oxygen dependency after 28 days, or after 36 weeks corrected gestation. However, the radiological changes develop during this period, usually following ventilation for hyaline membrane disease.
- Stages of bronchopulmonary dysplasia

Stage	Time	CXR appearance
1	<4 days	similar to hyaline membrane disease
2	4–10 days	complete opacification with air bronchograms or diffuse opacities
3	10–20 days	'bubbly' lungs : rounded lucencies surrounded by coarse linear densities
4	>1 month	as above with emphysematous change

- There may be complete radiological resolution over months or years in some cases. Others may have retained linear densities and upper lobe emphysema.

CLINICAL HOT LIST

- Chronic lung disease is seen following ventilation of the premature neonate. There is an increased incidence due to improved survival of very low birth weight infants.
- Aetiological factors include lung immaturity, barotrauma, oxygen toxicity, infection, patent ductus arteriosus, fluid overload, pulmonary interstitial emphysema and persistently abnormal surfactant. These lead to abnormal repair with fibroproliferative regeneration.

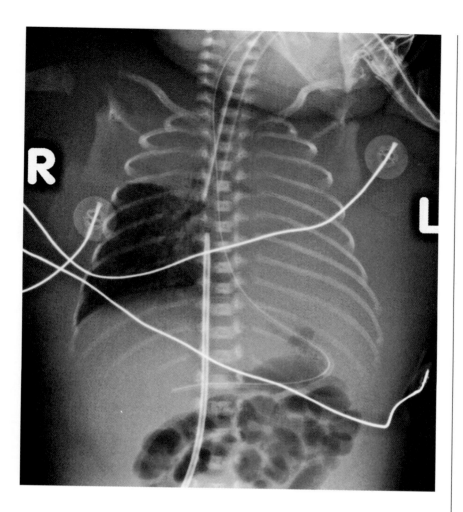

This 1 week old baby, born at 28 weeks' gestation, is being ventilated. His oxygen requirement has increased since re–intubation, and a repeat chest X–ray was requested.

1. What abnormalities are seen on the chest X-ray?
2. What is the appropriate next step?

ANSWERS

1. The tip of the endotracheal tube (ETT) lies too low, in the right main bronchus. This has resulted in collapse/consolidation of the entire left lung and right upper lobe. Only the right middle and lower lobe are aerated. (Note also the oedematous soft tissues due to fluid overload.)
2. The tube should be pulled back into a more satisfactory position.

RADIOLOGY HOT LIST

- The ETT may be inserted too far at intubation. The correct position for the ETT tip is halfway between the thoracic inlet and the carina (ideally at T1).
- Flexion of the baby's neck may cause a low-lying tube to slip into the right main bronchus. The right upper lobe bronchus may be occluded by the ETT (if the tip lies in the bronchus intermedius) causing collapse/consolidation of the right upper lobe.

CLINICAL HOT LIST

- Beware! Absent chest movement may indicate an oesophageal intubation. Asymmetrical chest movement and breath sounds should raise the suspicion of a malpositioned ETT.
- Always obtain a chest X-ray post intubation!

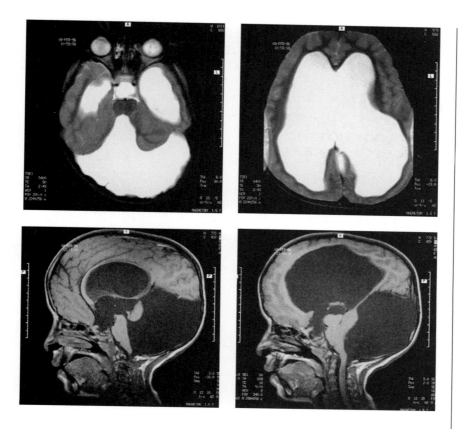

This 6 year old child was referred for assessment from abroad. He has a large head, mild developmental delay and convulsions dating from infancy.

MRI T1-weighted sagittal and T2-weighted axial images have been obtained.

1. What abnormality is demonstrated?
2. What is the diagnosis?

ANSWERS

1. There is cystic dilatation of the IVth ventricle, which fills the entire posterior fossa. There is agenesis of the cerebellar vermis, and elevation of the tentorium cerebelli. There is associated hydrocephalus.
2. Dandy–Walker malformation.

RADIOLOGY HOT LIST

- It is characterised by the absence/hypoplasia of the cerebellar vermis, and associated cerebellar hypoplasia.
- The IVth ventricle is grossly dilated, and the ensuing large posterior fossa cyst causes elevation of the tentorium.
- Hydrocephalus occurs secondary to atresia of the IVth ventricle foramina, aqueductal stenosis, or compression of the aqueduct by the cyst.
- It may be associated with neuromigrational disorders or agenesis of the corpus callosum.

CLINICAL HOT LIST

- Most cases are diagnosed on antenatal ultrasound. It may present later (uncommon in the UK) with a large head, developmental delay, ataxia and seizures.
- 50% have learning difficulties.
- It is usually sporadic, but occasionally associated with abnormalities of chromosome 9.
- It may be associated with other CNS malformations and midline facial and palate defects.
- Hydrocephalus may require ventriculo-peritoneal shunting.

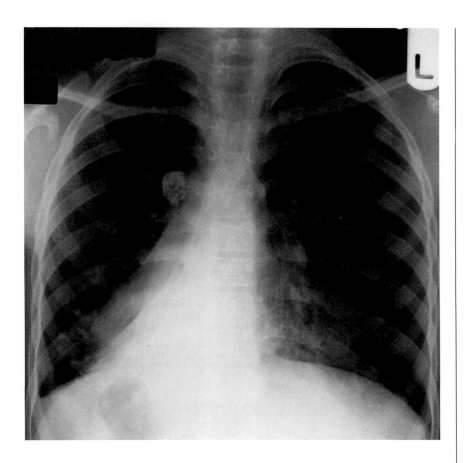

This 7 year old boy has a history of chronic cough with copious green sputum.

1. Name four abnormalities on the chest X-ray.
2. What is the diagnosis?

ANSWERS

1. There is dextrocardia and situs inversus (note right-sided stomach bubble). There is collapse of the right lower lobe (triangular density behind the heart) and consolidation medially at the left base. There are dilated bronchi with ring shadows in the left lower zone consistent with bronchiectasis. There is a calcified lymph node adjacent to the right-sided aortic arch.
2. Kartagener's syndrome with right lower lobe collapse and evidence of previous TB infection.

RADIOLOGY HOT LIST

- The combination of bronchiectasis and dextrocardia is highly suggestive of Kartagener's syndrome.
- Causes of childhood bronchiectasis:

Congenital	Dysmotile cilia syndrome (including Kartagener's), cystic fibrosis (abnormal secretions), structural defects of bronchi
Immunodeficiency	Hypogammaglobulinaemia, chronic granulomatous disease
Post-infectious	Measles, whooping cough, post-viral
Post-bronchial obstruction	Aspirated foreign body

CLINICAL HOT LIST

- Kartagener's syndrome consists of a clinical triad: situs inversus (50%), bronchiectasis and sinusitis. There may be deafness and infertility.
- There is mucociliary dysfunction (generalised deficiency of dynein arms of the cilia) affecting the respiratory and auditory epithelium, and sperm.
- Incidence 1 : 40 000, with a high familial incidence.
- There may be associated cardiac abnormalities (most commonly transposition of the great arteries).

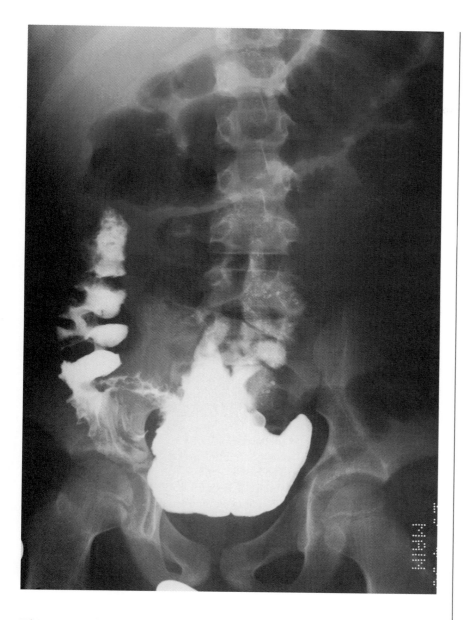

This 8 year old boy suffers from weight loss, abdominal pain and diarrhoea.

1. What investigation has been performed?
2. What abnormalities are seen?
3. What is the diagnosis?

ANSWERS

1. A barium follow-through, with contrast in the ileum, caecum, and ascending colon.
2. The terminal ileum is narrowed, the mucosa is irregular with nodular filling defects – a 'cobblestone' appearance. There is mucosal ulceration.
3. Crohn's disease.

RADIOLOGY HOT LIST

- Crohn's disease affects the small bowel in 80% of cases and the terminal ileum is the commonest site of disease.
- The 'cobblestone' pattern is due a combination of mucosal oedema and linear ulcers.
- Other features include thickened and distorted small bowel folds (earliest sign), 'rose thorn' ulcers and 'skip' lesions (intervening segments of normal bowel).
- Bowel loops may be widely separated (due to bowel wall thickening). Strictures and fistulae may be present.
- Other diseases affecting the terminal ileum include tuberculosis, *Yersinia* infection and lymphoma.

CLINICAL HOT LIST

- Incidence: 10–20 : 100 000 in the childhood population. Up to 40% of Crohn's disease presents before the age of 20.
- Presentation depends on the site of involvement (any part of the GI tract). The commonest presentation is with colicky abdominal pain, diarrhoea and poor growth. Subtle presentations may occur with oropharyngeal or perianal disease.
- Complications include fistulae, abscess formation and toxic megacolon.
- Management aims to induce and maintain remission of disease, and to restore normal growth. Strategies include steroids, sulphasalazine, immunosuppression and nutritional modification. Occasionally surgery is necessary, but is not curative.

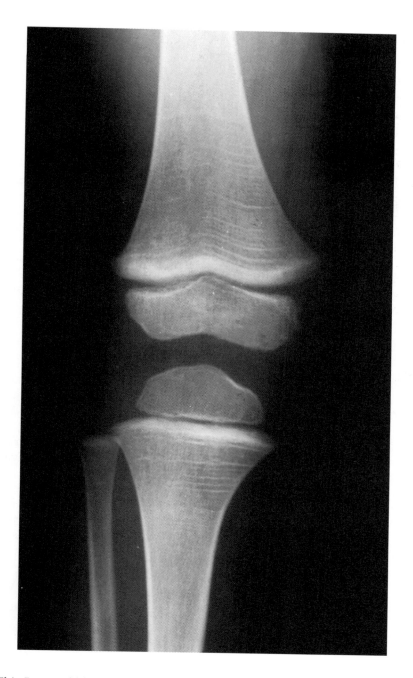

This 5 year old boy fell off his bike and required an X-ray of his right leg. An additional history was elicited of abdominal pain, loss of appetite and constipation.

1. What abnormality is seen on the X-ray of the right knee?
2. What is the diagnosis?

ANSWERS

1. The metaphyses of the femur, tibia and fibula are dense. There are growth arrest lines present.
2. Lead poisoning.

RADIOLOGY HOT LIST

- Lead affects bone growth in the metaphyseal region and leads to the appearance of dense metaphyseal bands. Later changes include modelling deformities.
- The abdominal film may show evidence of lead ingestion, with opacities in the bowel.
- In severe cases there may be widening of the sutures due to raised intracranial pressure.
- Other causes of dense metaphyseal bands include: normal infants (less than 3 years), healed rickets, osteopetrosis, hypothyroidism and hyper-vitaminosis D. They are not to be confused with growth arrest lines, which are usually thin sclerotic lines.

CLINICAL HOT LIST

- Lead poisoning is usually due to pica. It presents with irritability, abdominal pain, anorexia, failure to thrive and progressive deterioration in intelligence. If severe, drowsiness, convulsions and coma may occur.
- Raised blood lead levels confirm the diagnosis. There is anaemia with a characteristic blood film showing basophilic stippling.
- Management strategies include identification and removal of the source, and chelating agents (D-penicillamine). Sources include lead-based paints, old water pipes, lead shot, and some Indian eye make-up.

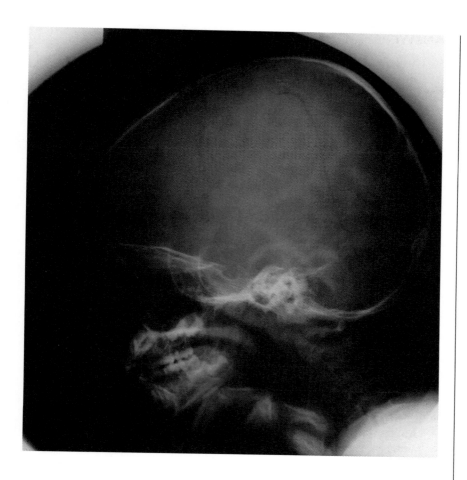

This 1 year old boy was admitted after a head injury at the crèche.

1. What does the lateral skull X-ray show?

ANSWERS

1. There is a lucent line across the parietal bone indicating a parietal skull fracture.

RADIOLOGY HOT LIST

- It is often difficult to differentiate between fractures, vascular markings and sutures.
- Fractures are usually straight lucent lines. Suture lines are interdigitated and in characteristic locations. Vascular markings usually have a tortuous and branching course.
- Depressed fractures usually appear as dense straight sclerotic lines.

FEATURES OF SKULL FRACTURES WHICH ARE SUSPICIOUS OF NON-ACCIDENTAL INJURY

1. Complex fractures involving both sides of skull.
2. Multiple fractures.
3. Widened fractures.
4. Fractures of different ages.
5. Depressed fractures, especially occipital.
6. Growing fractures (traumatic encephaloceles).

CLINICAL HOT LIST

- Simple skull fractures in accidental trauma have a very low risk of intracranial sequelae. They usually involve falls from short distances, which impart a linear force to the head.
- A detailed history is mandatory, as a simple skull fracture remains the most common injury seen in non–accidental head trauma.

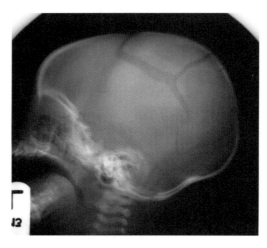

Skull fracture in non-accidental injury.

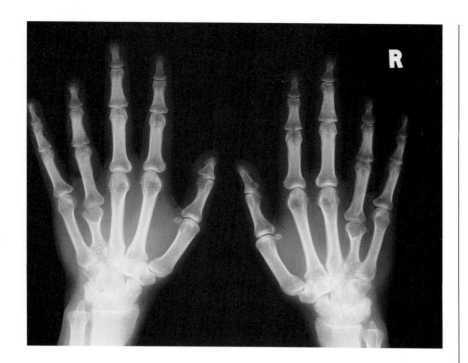

This is the X-ray of both hands of an 18 year old woman.

1. What abnormality is present?
2. What is the differential diagnosis?

ANSWERS

1. The fourth metacarpals are short – a tangential line drawn between the third and fifth metacarpal heads should intersect the fourth.
2. Pseudohypoparathyroidism, pseudopseudohypoparathyroidism, Turner's syndrome, idiopathic.

RADIOLOGY HOT LIST

- Pseudohypoparathyroidism and pseudopseudohypoparathyrodism have similar radiological findings including short metacarpals and metatarsals. CT may show basal ganglia calcification.
- Radiological findings in Turner's syndrome (45XO) include delayed epiphyseal fusion, osteoporosis (due to gonadal hormone deficiency), Madelung deformity, coarctation of the aorta, horseshoe kidney, lymph-oedema and cystic hygroma.
- Previous infarction (e.g. sickle cell anaemia) and growth plate injury can give a similar appearance, but is usually unilateral.

CLINICAL HOT LIST

- Pseudohypoparathyroidism is an inherited disorder of parathyroid hormone (PTH) end organ resistance. PTH production is normal. Clinical features include hypocalcaemia, short stature, obesity, and a variable degree of learning difficulties.
- Patients with pseudopseudohypoparathyroidism have the same phenotype, but without the metabolic abnormalities.

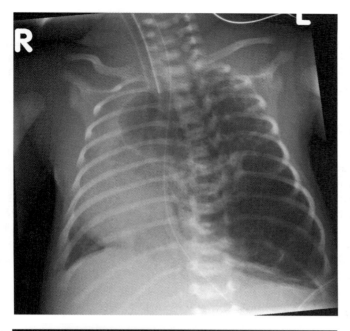

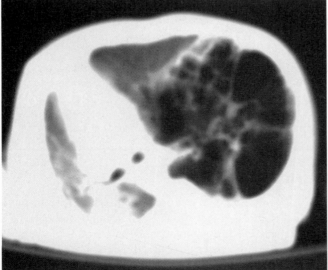

This baby was born at a specialist unit because of an antenatally diagnosed condition, and ventilated from birth.

1. What abnormalities are seen on the chest radiograph and CT scan?
2. What is the diagnosis?

ANSWERS

1. There are multiple large cystic spaces within the left hemithorax, which are causing mass effect with mediastinal shift. They do not extend below the diaphragm. The tip of the nasogastric tube lies below the diaphragm.
2. Congenital cystic adenomatoid malformation.

RADIOLOGY HOT LIST

- It is typically an expansile cystic mass (almost always unilateral) with well-defined margins. It is usually fluid filled initially, and becomes lucent as air replaces the fluid.
- Mediastinal shift, compression of adjacent lung and pulmonary hypoplasia are common. The abdominal viscera are normally sited.
- It is often detected antenatally, but may regress during the course of pregnancy and be barely detectable at birth. In this case postnatal imaging should include ultrasound or CT scan as the chest X-ray may appear normal.
- The differential diagnosis includes congenital diaphragmatic hernia, congenital lobar emphysema and a pneumothorax.

Type	Incidence	Appearance	Prognosis
Type 1	50%	Single/multiple large cysts >20 mm)	Excellent with surgical resection
Type 2	40%	Multiple cysts (5–20 mm)	Poor – may be associated with congenital abnormalities
Type 3	10%	Large solid mass with no macroscopic cysts	Poor – due to associated pulmonary hypoplasia

CLINICAL HOT LIST

- This is a congenital hamartomatous lesion, which communicates with the bronchial tree and has a normal arterial supply and venous drainage. The characteristic cystic appearance develops postnatally as air-trapping occurs within the abnormal pulmonary tissue.
- The lesion is associated with a high mortality: 25% are stillborn; 20% have other congenital abnormalities (cardiac, renal, chromosomal anomalies).
- Potential antenatal interventions include aspiration, cystoamniotic shunt and fetal lobectomy.
- There has been a recent increase in surgical excision of small and large lesions because of the small risk of malignant transformation.

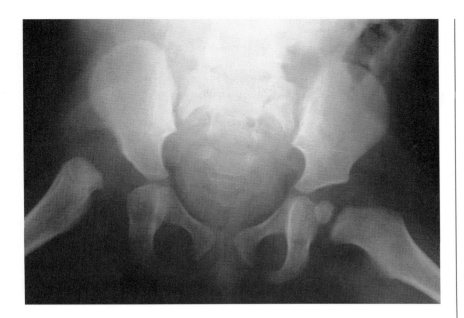

A 9 month old baby has been noticed to have asymmetrical thigh creases.

1. What does the plain X-ray of the pelvis show?
2. What is the diagnosis?
3. Name three associated factors.

ANSWERS

1. The right femur is displaced upwards and laterally. The right femoral capital epiphysis is not seen, and the acetabulum on this side is poorly developed (with steep angulation of the acetabular roof).
2. Developmental dysplasia of the right hip, resulting in dislocation.
3. Family history, breech position in utero, other congenital limb abnormalities, oligohydraminos.

RADIOLOGY HOT LIST

- The plain radiograph is useful after the femoral capital epiphysis has ossified (4–6 months).
- Prior to this, ultrasound is the investigation of choice (no radiation and good visualisation of the cartilaginous femoral head and acetabulum). Ultrasound demonstrates the degree of coverage of the head by the acetabulum, and the angle of the acetabular roof.
- There is a spectrum of ultrasound findings from mild dysplasia to frank dislocation. Most mildly dysplastic hips resolve on follow-up.

CLINICAL HOT LIST

- Incidence 1 : 100 at birth, 1 : 1000 at 1 year, F > M, bilateral in 10%.
- There is a spectrum from dislocatable to frank dislocation at rest.
- The clinical manifestations depend on age: asymmetrical thigh creases, delayed walking, Trendelenburg dip and waddling gait.
- Management depends on age at detection: persistent dislocation requires reduction and splinting or Pavlik harness for 3–6 months. After 6 months of age, an abduction plaster for 3 months or open reduction/femoral osteotomy may be required.

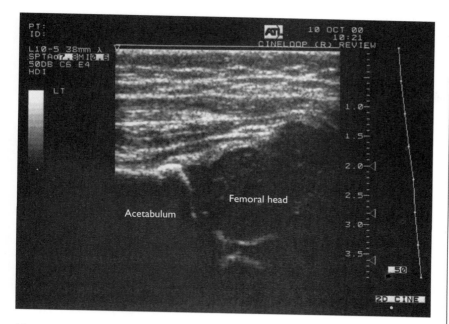

(a)

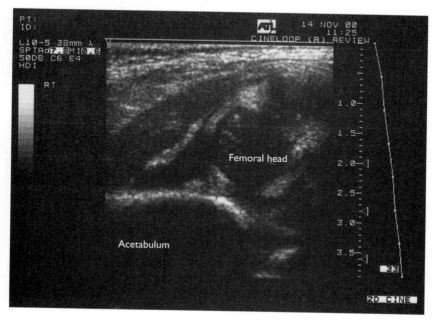

(b)

Ultrasound images of: (a) normal hip and (b) dislocated hip.

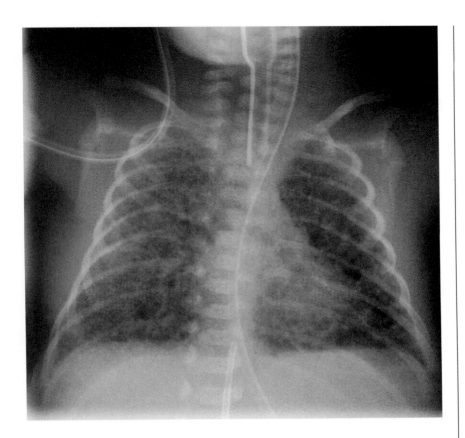

This 9 day old neonate, born at 28 weeks' gestation, was ventilated for hyaline membrane disease.

1. What abnormality is seen on the chest radiograph?
2. What is the diagnosis?

ANSWERS

1. The lungs are hyperinflated (nine posterior ribs visible and flattened diaphragms). Multiple, small, cystic air spaces are seen throughout both lungs. There is no pneumothorax present. There is an endotracheal tube, a nasogastric tube and a UAC in situ.
2. Pulmonary interstitial emphysema (PIE).

RADIOLOGY HOT LIST

- PIE is a radiological diagnosis in an ill, ventilated neonate, usually with HMD, occasionally sepsis or meconium aspiration.
- The changes may be bilateral, but are often unilateral with mediastinal shift towards the unaffected side.
- Pneumothorax and pneumomediastinum are frequent complications.

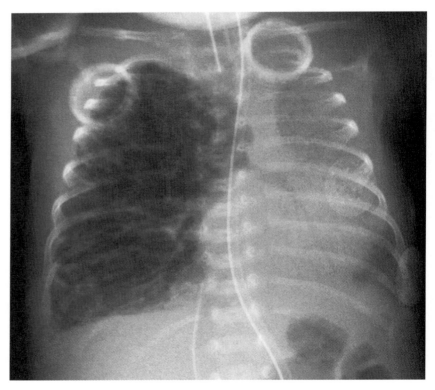

CXR showing unilateral PIE.

CLINICAL HOT LIST

- PIE occurs predominantly as a consequence of mechanical ventilatation of neonates. Small airways rupture, causing air to leak into the broncho-vascular sheaths.
- Changes of PIE occur within the first 2 weeks of life. Early presentation is associated with a worse prognosis, and is indicative of more severe underlying pulmonary disease.
- PIE is associated with high ventilator pressures, misplaced endotracheal tube and other air leaks. It may lead to pulmonary hypertension and right-to-left ductal shunting. There is a high incidence of subsequent chronic lung disease.
- Management includes keeping pressures to a minimum and decompression stategies, e.g. nursing with the affected side down, pleurotomy, and selective intubation.

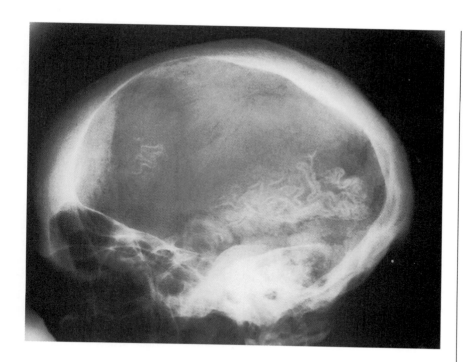

This 16 year old boy is under follow-up for recurrent seizures. He has a 'birth mark' on the right side of his face, and a left hemiparesis.

1. List two abnormalities demonstrated on the lateral skull X-ray.
2. What is the diagnosis?

ANSWERS

1. There is serpiginous, tram-track calcification in the frontal and occipital region. The skull vault is markedly thickened.
2. Sturge–Weber syndrome.

RADIOLOGY HOT LIST

- Classical radiological appearances include gyriform intracranial calcification, cortical hemiatrophy with a thickened skull vault on the side of the angioma, and dilated ventricles with choroid plexus hypertrophy.
- Tram-track calcification following the contours of the gyri is not usually seen on plain radiographs until the age of 2 years. CT scans may show superficial cortical calcification at an earlier stage.

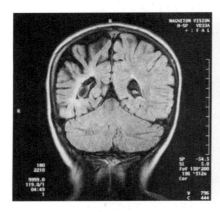 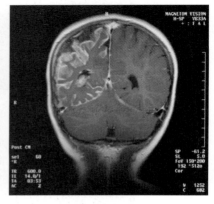

Pre- and post-enhancement T1-weighted MRI showing cortical atrophy of the right parietal and occipital lobes, and right meningeal enhancement. There is choroid plexus hypertrophy in the right lateral ventricle. There is some minor thickening of the right side of the vault.

CLINICAL HOT LIST

- A congenital vascular anomaly involving the eye, skin and brain.
- It is characterised by a port wine naevus of the face in the distribution of the trigeminal nerve (face and forehead), with a venous angioma of the ipsilateral cerebral meninges. These are thin-walled vessels within the pia mater.
- Clinical features include mental retardation, seizures (>90%), contra-lateral hemiparesis and hemiatrophy and ipsilateral glaucoma.
- Management strategies include antiepileptic therapy and occasionally neurosurgical procedures for intractable epilepsy.

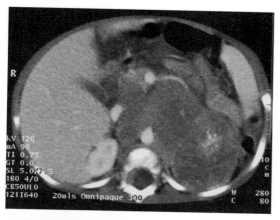

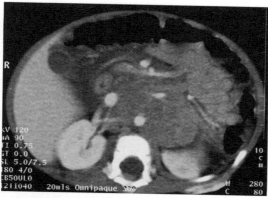

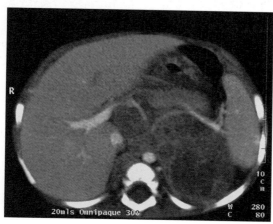

This 18-month old boy presented with fever and weight loss. On examination, he was anaemic and had a palpable abdominal mass.

1. What abnormalities are shown on the contrast-enhanced CT scan of the abdomen?
2. What is the diagnosis?

ANSWERS

1. There is a large left suprarenal mass containing amorphous calcification and low-attenuation areas (consistent with central necrosis). It encases the aorta and coeliac axis, which is stretched anteriorly. The inferior vena cava (IVC) is displaced to the left whilst the left kidney is displaced inferiorly.
2. Neuroblastoma.

RADIOLOGY HOT LIST

- Neuroblastoma is the commonest extracranial malignant tumour of childhood.
- It arises in the abdomen in 60%, usually in the adrenal gland. 65% of patients have metastatic disease at presentation (bone, spinal canal, lymph nodes, lung and liver).
- Ultrasound will confirm the presence and location of an abdominal mass but CT/MRI is required for staging.
- Nuclear medicine scans (MIBG and bone scans) are performed to detect distant metastases, and to evaluate response to chemotherapy.
- Features distinguishing Wilm's tumour from neuroblastoma:

Wilms'	Neuroblastoma
Intrinsic renal mass	external compression/displacement of kidney
10% bilateral	unilateral but usually crosses midline
<10% contain calcification	85% contain calcification
Displaces vessels. Renal vein invasion in 5–10%	vessel encasement

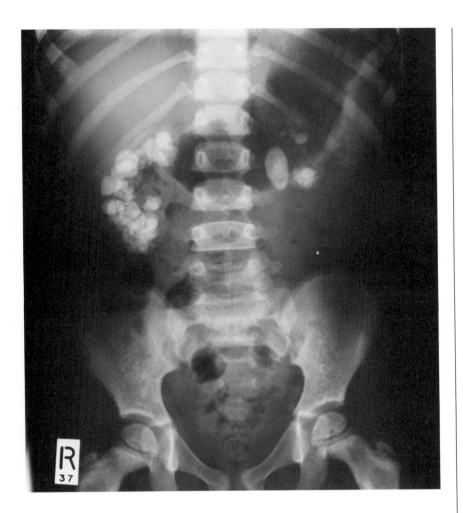

This 4 year old girl with an inherited condition has renal failure.

1. What does the plain abdominal X-ray show?
2. List four possible causes?

ANSWERS

1. There is bilateral nephrocalcinosis (widespread calcification throughout the renal parenchyma) and there is a large calculus in the region of the left renal pelvis. The metaphyses show changes of renal osteodystrophy.
2. Medullary sponge kidney, renal tubular acidosis, hyperparathyroidism and hyperoxaluria. This child has primary hyperoxaluria.

RADIOLOGY HOT LIST

- Nephrocalcinosis is the deposition of calcium salts in the renal parenchyma. It is subdivided into cortical nephrocalcinosis (5%, peripheral calcification sparing medullary pyramids) and medullary nephrocalcinosis (95%, calcification of medullary pyramids).
- The calcification occurs in the parenchyma of the kidney, as opposed to the collecting system (as with renal calculi). Renal calculi may also occur in some of the conditions causing nephrocalcinosis.

	Causes
Medullary nephrocalcinosis	any cause of hypercalcaemia/ hypercalcuria (hyperparathyroidism, hypervitaminosis D), renal tubular acidosis, medullary sponge kidney and hyperoxaluria
Cortical nephrocalcinosis	chronic glomerulonephritis, cortical necrosis, primary hyperoxaluria and Alport's syndrome

CLINICAL HOT LIST

- Primary hyperoxaluria is a rare autosomal recessive condition which causes diffuse deposition of oxalate in the kidneys, heart, lung, spleen and bone marrow.
- Presentation occurs at <5 years old, with early death occurring in childhood.
- Secondary hyperoxaluria occurs where there is disruption of the bile acid enterocirculation. Causes include ileal resection and Crohn's disease.

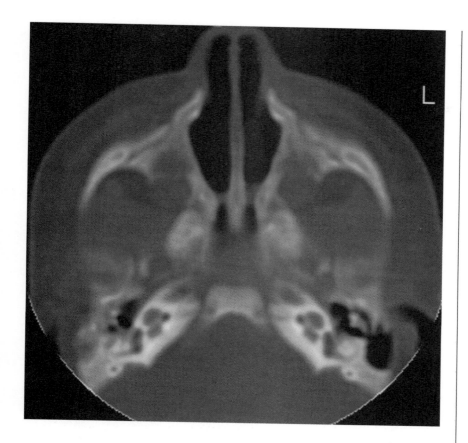

This 1 day old term baby has tachypnoea and cyanosis during feeding. The midwives are unable to pass a nasogastric tube to facilitate top-up feeds.

1. What does the CT scan through the nasopharynx show?
2. What is the diagnosis?

ANSWERS

1. There are membranous septa occluding the posterior aspect of the nasal air passages bilaterally. The lateral walls of the nasal cavity are deviated medially.

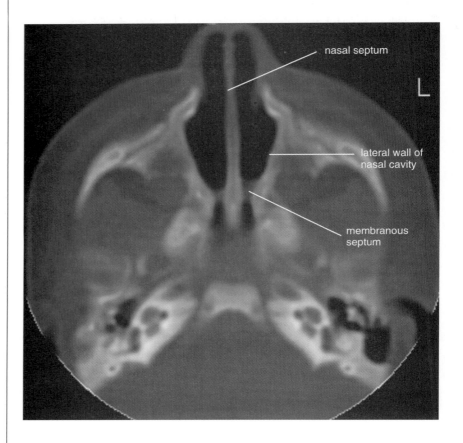

nasal septum

L

lateral wall of nasal cavity

membranous septum

2. Bilateral membranous choanal atresia.

RADIOLOGY HOT LIST

- The occlusion may be bony (85%) or membranous (15%).
- A CT scan of the nasal airways (fine cuts) is the examination of choice – but the baby needs suction before the examination to ensure that retained secretions are not misinterpreted as membranous septa.

CLINICAL HOT LIST

- Incidence 1 : 8000, unilateral more common than bilateral. 50% are associated with CHARGE syndrome (**C**oloboma, **H**eart disease, choanal **A**tresia, **R**etarded growth, **G**enital hypoplasia, **E**ar abnormalities). There is also an association with Treacher–Collins syndrome.
- It usually presents with apnoea, cyanosis, respiratory distress and feeding difficulties in a neonate. Unilateral atresia may present later with milder symptoms or nasal discharge.
- Babies are obligatory nose-breathers until 3 months of age, unless they are crying. These babies may therefore be pink when crying and distressed/dusky at rest.
- The diagnosis may be suspected by the inability to pass a nasogastric tube.
- The airway may require protection (oral airway or intubation) prior to definitive surgery.

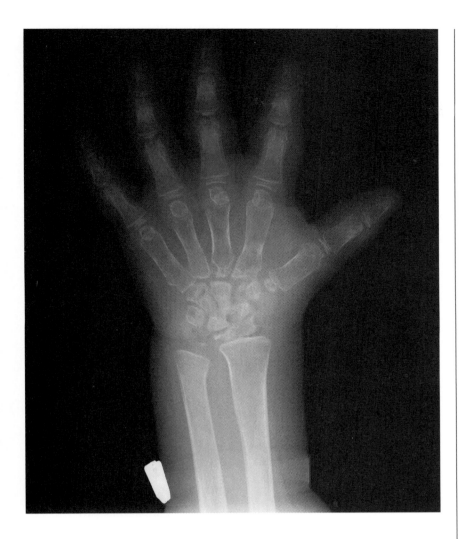

This 4 year old boy has a painful left wrist.

1. What does the X-ray show?
2. What is the diagnosis?

ANSWERS

1. There is soft tissue swelling around the wrist. The bones are osteopenic. The carpal bones are small and irregular, with multiple erosions. There are further erosions of the bases of the second, third and fourth metacarpals and of many of the small joints. There is loss of the joint space at the radiocarpal and intercarpal joints.
2. Juvenile idiopathic arthritis (JIA).

RADIOLOGY HOT LIST

- The earliest signs in the wrist include periarticular osteopenia and soft tissue swelling. Later changes include erosions, periosteal reactions, joint space loss, and joint destruction.
- Spinal changes include diffuse ankylosis of the posterior articular joints (especially in the cervical spine) and atlanto-axial subluxation.
- Hyperaemia of the affected joints may cause overgrowth of the epiphyses with premature closure of the growth plates (and therefore bone shortening).
- Gadolinium-enhanced MRI scans can detect synovial hypertrophy and acute synovitis.

CLINICAL HOT LIST

- JIA has an onset below the age of 16. Symptoms must be present for more than 3 months
- Three clinical categories:

Systemic onset	10%, M = F	swinging fever, splenomegaly, lymphadenopathy, rash; arthritis may initially be absent
Polyarticular	40%, F > M	five or more joints affected, symmetrical involvement of small joints of hands and feet, as well as large joints; 10% are rheumatoid factor positive
Pauciarticular	50%, early onset F > M, late onset M > F	< 5 large joints affected, systemic features usually absent; associated with uveitis; late onset associated with HLA-B27 and spinal disease (similar to ankylosing spondylosis)

- JIA requires multidisciplinary management including drugs (NSAIDS, steroids, methotrexate), physiotherapy, occupational therapy and psychological support.

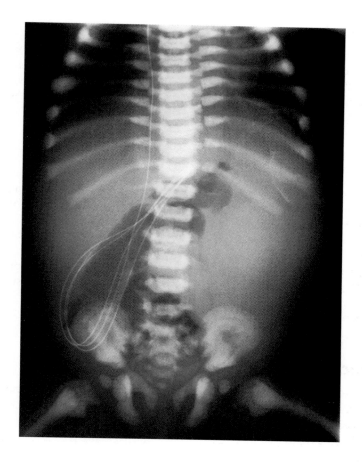

This 6 month old baby has a rare inherited disorder. On examination he has hepatosplenomegaly.

1. What abnormalities are seen on the X-ray?
2. What is the diagnosis?

ANSWERS

1. The bones are diffusely sclerotic, with obliteration of the normal trabecular pattern. There is a 'bone-within-a-bone' appearance best appreciated in the pelvis and proximal femora. There is displacement of the bowel gas by an enlarged liver and spleen.
2. Osteopetrosis (Albers–Schönberg disease)

RADIOLOGY HOT LIST

- A characteristic finding is diffuse osteosclerosis with cortical thickening and medullary encroachment. The bones appear dense with loss of the normal trabecular pattern. The 'bone-within-bone' appearance is classical.
- Though appearing sclerotic, the bones are actually brittle and weak – look for pathological fractures, which usually heal with exuberant callus formation.
- Osteosclerosis causes obliteration of the paranasal sinuses, mastoid air cells and skull base foramina.

CLINICAL HOT LIST

- This is a rare hereditary disorder with both recessive and dominant inheritance – the latter being clinically less severe.
- There is a failure of osteoclast resorption causing persistence of the cartilaginous and calcified bone matrix. The bones are abnormally sclerotic but structurally weak.
- Obliteration of the medullary cavity causes marrow depression with subsequent anaemia, leucocytopenia, and thrombocytopenia. Extra-medullary haemopoiesis leads to hepatosplenomegaly.
- Bony overgrowth causes narrowing of the neural foramina resulting in cranial nerve palsies. Optic atrophy and deafness are common findings in the recessive form.
- In the recessive form survival beyond middle age is uncommon and death is usually due to haemorrhage, recurrent infection or leukaemia.
- Bone marrow transplantation is potentially curative.

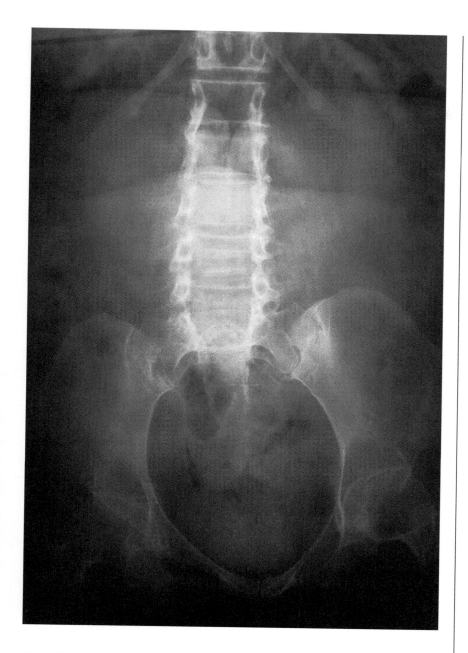

This 18 year old girl is paraplegic, with urinary and faecal incontinence.

1. What does the X-ray of the lumbar spine show?
2. What is the diagnosis?

ANSWERS

1. The posterior elements of the lumbar spine are absent (absent laminae and spinous processes) with a widened spinal canal. Note the widening of the interpedicular distance.
2. Spina bifida.

RADIOLOGY HOT LIST

- Remember to assess the spine on a plain film of the abdomen! Identify the pedicles, laminae and spinous processes – if these are absent, or incompletely fused, a diagnosis of spinal dysraphism can be made.
- The diagnosis is often made by antenatal ultrasound (complex mass seen outside spinal canal with separation of the posterior laminae).
- There is a high incidence of associated hydrocephalus (usually detected antenatally).
- There may be other CNS abnormalities including Arnold–Chiari malformation, intraspinal dermoid and lipoma, tethered cord and diastematomyelia. These can be further assessed with MRI. Ultrasound can be used to assess the spine in young babies.

CLINICAL HOT LIST

- Spinal dysraphism is a spectrum of disorders ranging from mildly deficient lumbar spinous processes (spina bifida occulta) to an open defect with exposed abnormal spinal cord and CSF leakage (spina bifida cystica).
- Clinical manifestations depend on the site and extent of the lesion. There may be complete loss of motor, sensory and reflex function below the affected level. Involvement of the sacral roots leads to bowel and bladder dysfunction.
- Neurosurgical repair aims to achieve a water-tight closure of the defect without worsening the neurological status. Ventricular shunting may be required for hydrocephalus.
- Multidisciplinary managment should include neurosurgical, orthopaedic and urological input as well as physiotherapy and occupational therapy assessment.

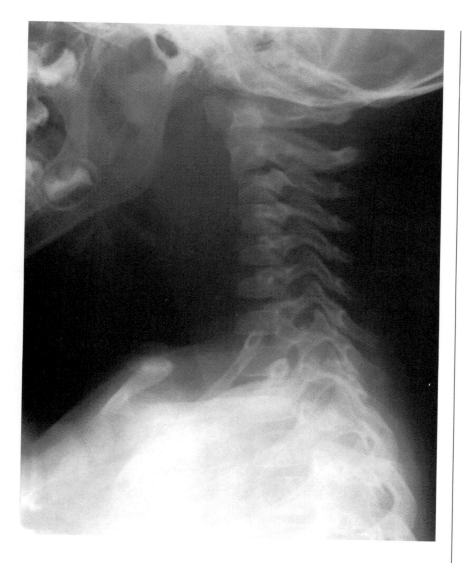

This 2 year old boy has fever and dysphagia.

1. What abnormality is seen on the lateral X-ray of the neck?
2. What is the diagnosis?

ANSWERS

1. There is swelling of the prevertebral soft tissues with anterior displacement of the trachea. There is loss of the normal cervical lordosis but the bones appear normal.
2. Retropharyngeal abscess.

RADIOLOGY HOT LIST

- Swelling of the prevertebral soft tissues implies infection or haemorrhage. In a child the thickness of the normal prevertebral soft tissues is 3–5 mm between C1 and C4 (2–3 mm in an adult) and the width of the vertebral body below C4.
- There may be reversal of the normal cervical lordosis as the head is held in an abnormal position. Erosion of bone or disc height reduction indicates an underlying osteomyelitis or discitis.
- Gas or an air–fluid level in the retropharyngeal tissues is highly suggestive of an abscess.
- A contrast-enhanced CT scan will confirm the diagnosis in equivocal cases and define the superior and inferior mediastinal extent.
- The differential diagnosis includes haematoma, lymphadenopathy, and (rarely) neoplasm (rhabdomyosarcoma).

CLINICAL HOT LIST

- Rare infection of the posterior pharyngeal wall occurring in young children and babies.
- Aetiology: upper respiratory tract infection, extension of suppurative cervical lymphadenitis, or perforating injury of the pharynx or oesophagus.
- It presents with fever, drooling and with the head held back due to airway obstruction. Important differential diagnoses include epiglottitis and tonsillitis.
- Typical organisms: *staphylococcus*, *streptococcus*, mixed flora.

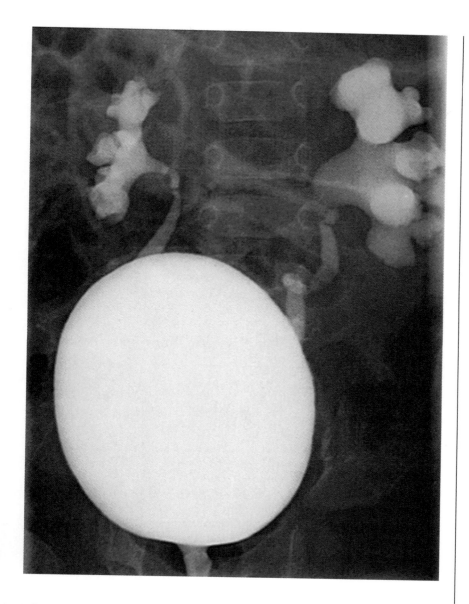

This 4 month old girl had been treated for a urinary tract infection. A micturating cystourethrogram was performed as part of her investigations.

1. What abnormalities are seen?
2. What is the diagnosis?

ANSWERS

1. Contrast has refluxed into dilated collecting systems and ureters bilaterally. The renal calyces are clubbed.
2. Bilateral vesicoureteric reflux (VUR).

RADIOLOGY HOT LIST

- There is still controversy over the strategy for investigation of urinary tract infection, with debate over the choice of investigation used to detect reflux and the age group which should be investigated. There is thus local variation in practice.
- A contrast MCUG is recommended in boys where visualisation of the urethra is important in order to exclude posterior urethral valves.
- When possible, girls can have a direct nuclear medicine cystogram, as images of the urethra are not required. Beyond the age of 3, most children can micturate on request. Nuclear medicine studies then become the investigation of choice, with a reduction in radiation dose, and a more pleasant experience for all concerned.
- Grading of reflux:

Grade	
1	Reflux to ureter, but not kidney
2	Reflux into non-dilated ureter, pelvis, and calyces
3	Reflux to calyces with mild dilatation
4	Reflux to calyces, with moderate dilatation and clubbed calyces
5	Gross dilatation and tortuous ureters

CLINICAL HOT LIST

- VUR must be considered in a child with a UTI, as there is an important association with renal scarring, hypertension and chronic renal failure. Most cases of VUR resolve spontaneously.
- Management (prophylactic antibiotics, frequent voiding, treatment of constipation) aims to prevent renal scarring by prevention of UTI. Parental vigilance for UTI symptoms, and regular assessment of renal growth and possible scarring are essential.
- Surgical management, including ureteric reimplantation, is reserved for failure of medical management, complex abnormalities and obstruction.

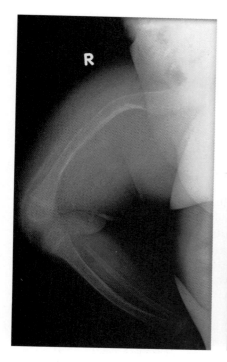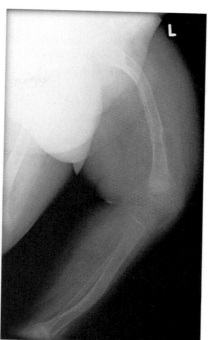

This 18 month old girl has had multiple admissions after minor trauma.

1. What do the X-rays of the legs show?
2. What is the diagnosis?

ANSWERS

1. The bones are osteopenic with cortical thinning and modelling deformities (markedly bowed). There is a breach in the cortex of the left femoral shaft associated with a periosteal reaction indicating a recent fracture.
2. Osteogenesis imperfecta.

RADIOLOGY HOT LIST

- Radiographic features of osteogenesis imperfecta include generalised cortical thinning, with gracile bones. The proximal humeri and femora may be expanded. There are usually bowing deformities present.
- Fractures are common, and they may heal with exuberant callus formation. Operative interventions (osteotomy and internal pinning) are frequent.
- There may be Wormian (intrasutural) bones in the skull, and a thin calvarium. Kyphoscoliosis and vertebral scalloping are a common finding in the spine. The pelvis may show protrusio acetabulae.

CLINICAL HOT LIST

- These are a group of inherited disorders of defective production of type I collagen. The management strategy involves prevention of fractures, orthopaedic management, and early mobilisation.

Type	Inheritance	Clinical manifestations
I	AD	commonest form, with pathological fractures as a toddler, blue sclerae, hypotonia, hypermobility, deafness, abnormal teeth
II	new dominant mutation	multiple intrauterine fractures with death in utero
III	AD/AR	multiple fractures from infancy, severe progressive skeletal deformities, kyphoscoliosis, chest deformities, premature death from respiratory failure
IV	AD	bone disease similar to type I, but manifestations are less severe than types II and III

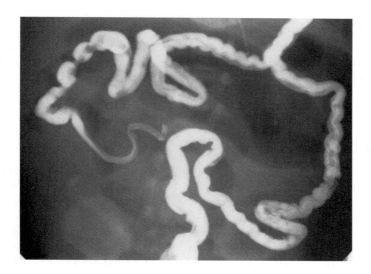

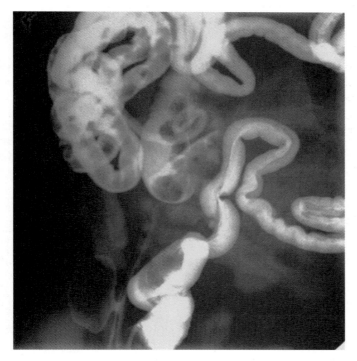

This 3 day old baby was brought to A&E with bilious vomiting, abdominal distension and failure to pass meconium. The plain abdominal radiograph shows multiple dilated loops of bowel. A contrast enema was performed.

1. List three abnormalities demonstrated on the enema.
2. What is the diagnosis?
3. What is the associated condition?

ANSWERS

1. There is a narrow calibre empty colon (microcolon). There are dilated loops of small bowel. The second image shows the distal ileum containing large filling defects, which are meconium plugs.
2. Meconium ileus.
3. Cystic fibrosis.

RADIOLOGY HOT LIST

- A contrast enema is the investigation of choice in low bowel obstruction.
- In this case, contrast refluxes back into the terminal ileum, which appears larger than the colon. The ileum contains multiple rounded filling defects due to masses of inspissated meconium.
- Distinguish this appearance from meconium plug syndrome, which is a functional motility disorder of the bowel and not associated with cystic fibrosis. A contrast enema in this condition shows a large filling defect in the rectum and colon due to a long meconium cast.
- Both conditions may be treated with a therapeutic enema to relieve the obstruction (successful in 50% of cases of meconium ileus; the other 50% will require surgery).

CLINICAL HOT LIST

- Meconium ileus is almost always associated with cystic fibrosis. The meconium is thick and viscid, occluding small bowel and not passing distally. The associated microcolon is of normal length and orientation but narrow calibre. It is unused, containing no (or very little) meconium.
- 10% of cystic fibrosis patients present with neonatal intestinal obstruction.
- Meconium plug syndrome is a neonatal functional motility disorder.

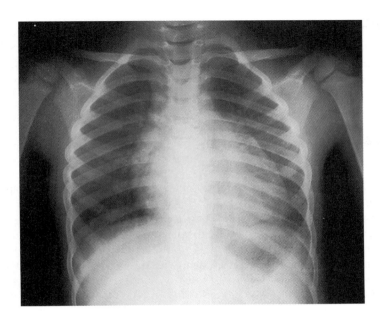

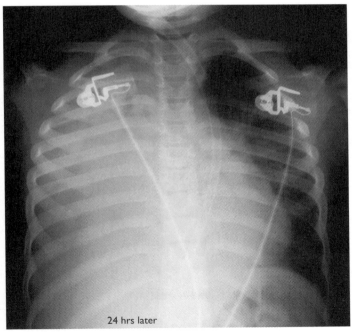

24 hrs later

This 8 year old Afro-Caribbean girl was admitted to the ward with chest pain, low oxygen saturations and respiratory distress. She has an underlying haematological condition. These chest X-rays were taken 24 hours apart.

1. What change is seen over the 24 hour interval between the X-rays?
2. What is the most likely diagnosis?

ANSWERS

1. The heart is enlarged on both films. The lungs are initially clear. However, after 24 hours there is opacification of the right hemithorax. There is also increased density behind the heart on the left, which contains an air bronchogram. This implies consolidation in the entire right lung and left lower lobe.
2. Acute sickle chest syndrome.

RADIOLOGY HOT LIST

- Sickle chest syndrome comprises changes of pulmonary infarction and subsequent consolidation.
- The rapid widespread change is suggestive of sickle chest syndrome. The differential diagnosis for consolidation in sickle cell disease is pneumococcal pneumonia, which classically causes lobar consolidation.
- Cardiomegaly may occur due to haemosiderotic cardiomyopathy (repeated transfusions causing iron overload) or high output cardiac failure.

CLINICAL HOT LIST

- Sickle cell disease is a chronic haemolytic anaemia with intermittent symptoms due to infarction, sequestration and infection. These may be precipitated by the cold, infection, dehydration and acidosis.
- Clinical presentations:

Dactylitis	infantile presentation affecting hands and feet
Splenic sequestration	rapid life-threatening hypovolaemic shock caused by extensive red cell trapping in spleen
Painful crisis	widespread microvascular occlusion usually in long bones or back
Aplastic crisis	reticulocyte failure due to parvovirus or folate deficiency
Neurological crisis	acute stroke, intracerebral sickling
Infection	bacteraemia or osteomyelitis secondary to *pneumococcus*, *haemophilus*, or *salmonella*
Chest syndrome	pulmonary infarction

- Management strategies: parental education, penicillin prophylaxis and avoidance of crisis precipitants.
- Management of an acute crisis includes oxygen, hydration, analgesia and antibiotics. Exchange transfusion may be required for chest and neurological crises. Immediate transfusion is indicated for splenic sequestration.

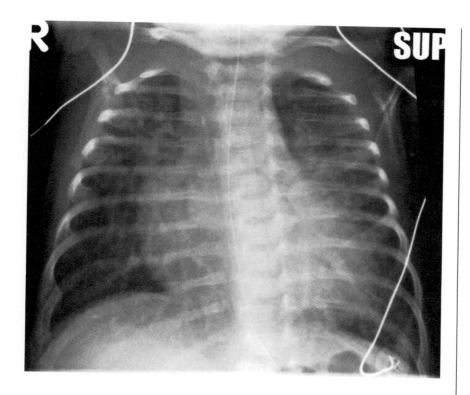

This 2 month old boy with Down's syndrome has been short of breath at rest since birth. On examination he is not cyanosed.

1. What does the chest X-ray show?
2. What is the most likely diagnosis?

ANSWERS

1. There is cardiomegaly with pulmonary plethora. No pleural effusion seen.
2. Left-to-right shunt, most likely an atrioventricular septal defect (AVSD) in a child with Down's syndrome.

RADIOLOGY HOT LIST

- Cardiomegaly is defined as a cardiothoracic ratio (CTR) > 0.5 on a PA chest X-ray. As most paediatric chest X-rays are taken AP, measuring the CTR is not always accurate. Gross enlargement can usually be identified.
- Causes of cardiomegaly include: congenital heart disease, congestive cardiac failure, pericardial effusion, myocarditis and cardiomyopathy.
- Acyanotic congenital heart disease with increased pulmonary vascularity is most commonly caused by a left-to-right shunt, which may occur at different anatomical sites.
- Causes of acyanotic congenital heart disease:

Increased vascularity	left to right shunts: ventriculoseptal defect (VSD), atrial septal defect (ASD), AVSD, patent ductus arteriosus
Normal/reduced vascularity	pulmonary stenosis, aortic stenosis, coarctation of the aorta

CLINICAL HOT LIST

- Congenital heart disease occurs in 40% of babies with Down's syndrome (usually AVSD, ostium primum). Many cases are inoperable and develop early pulmonary hypertension and intractable heart failure.

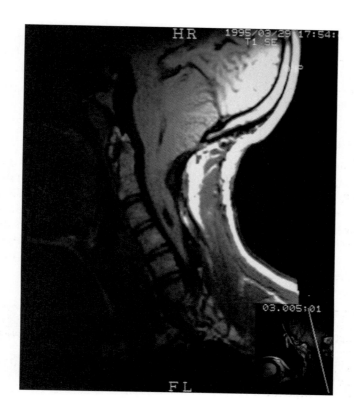

This 14 year old girl has a lumbar myelomeningocele.

1. What abnormalities are seen on the (T1-weighted) midline sagittal MRI scan?
2. What is the diagnosis?

ANSWERS

1. The cerebellar tonsils and vermis are herniated through the foramen magnum, with an elongated and caudally displaced IVth ventricle. There is a syrinx in the cervical cord.
2. Arnold–Chiari type II malformation.

RADIOLOGY HOT LIST

- The characteristic radiological findings in Arnold–Chiari type II malformation are hindbrain dygenesis with a caudally displaced IVth ventricle and brainstem, and herniation of the cerebellar tonsils through the foramen magnum.
- The degree of abnormality can vary widely from patient to patient.
- Associations:

Spinal anomalies	lumbar myelomeningoceles (>95%), syringomyelia
Supratentorial anomalies	obstructive hydrocephalus, dysgenesis of the corpus callosum, excessive cortical gyration

- Arnold–Chiari type I (mild herniation of the cerebellar tonsils) is a frequent isolated finding, often of little clinical significance and without associated supratentorial abnormalities.

CLINICAL HOT LIST

- Clinical manifestations include hydrocephalus, lower limb spasticity, upper limb weakness, Erb's palsy, neck pain, lower cranial nerve palsies (due to downward displacement of medulla) and respiratory abnormalities (brainstem compression).
- Neurosurgical management may be required to decompress the foramen magnum.

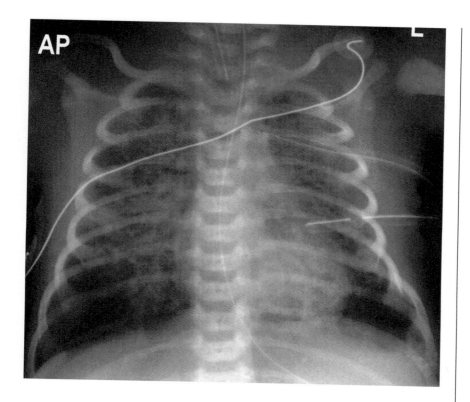

This term baby was admitted to the neonatal unit after an emergency Caesarean section for fetal distress.

1. What abnormalities are seen on the chest radiograph?
2. What is the most likely diagnosis?

ANSWERS

1. The lungs are hyperinflated with flattened hemidiaphragms. There is bilateral, asymmetrical opacification of the lung fields with coarse patchy infiltrates. There are areas of air trapping at both lung bases. Two inter-costal drains are present in the left hemithorax, but no pneumothorax is seen.
2. Meconium aspiration syndrome.

RADIOLOGY HOT LIST

- Meconium aspiration causes obstruction of the airways resulting in hyperinflation and areas of atelectasis and air trapping. Radiographic appearances depend on the severity of the aspiration.
- Look for pneumothorax and pneumomediastinum (seen in 25% of cases).
- Radiographic appearances may be indistinguishable from neonatal pneumonia and pulmonary haemorrhage.

CLINICAL HOT LIST

- This disorder occurs because of fetal asphyxia in term and postmature neonates.

Meconium	Pulmonary effects
Highly viscous	ball–valve effect causes air trapping
Chemical irritant	pneumonitis
Opposes surfactant	reduces lung compliance
Associated with chorioamnionitis	pneumonia

- A major complication is persistent pulmonary hypertension. This may be unresponsive to conventional measures, necessitating high frequency oscillation ventilation, nitric oxide or extracorporeal membrane oxidation (ECMO).
- It is associated with hypoxic ischaemic encephalopathy and renal failure (secondary to asphyxia).

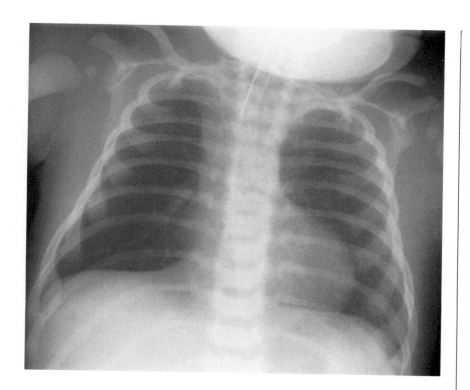

This one day old baby is cyanotic.

1. What does the chest X-ray show?
2. What is the diagnosis?

ANSWERS

1. There is a boot-shaped heart. The cardiac apex is elevated (right ventricular hypertrophy) and the pulmonary bay is concave due to a hypoplastic main pulmonary artery. The lungs are relatively oligaemic. The endotracheal tube is in a satisfactory position.
2. Tetralogy of Fallot.

RADIOLOGY HOT LIST

- Tetralogy of Fallot has a typical radiographic appearance due to right ventricular hypertrophy and underdevelopment of the main pulmonary artery. There may be a right-sided aortic arch in 25%.
- Evaluate the pulmonary vascularity on the chest X-ray: this will narrow the differential diagnosis in the assessment of cyanotic congenital heart disease.
- CXR appearances in cyanotic congenital heart disease:

Pulmonary vascularity	Causes
Increased	Transposition of the great arteries, truncus arteriosus, total anomalous pulmonary venous drainage, single ventricle
Decreased with normal heart size	Tetralogy of Fallot
Decreased with cardiomegaly	Ebstein's anomaly, pulmonary atresia, tricuspid atresia

CLINICAL HOT LIST

- Fallot's tetralogy is the commonest congenital cyanotic cardiac lesion (6% of all congenital heart malformations).
- The tetralogy comprises a ventricular septal defect, pulmonary stenosis, overriding aorta and right ventricular hypertrophy.
- It presents with cyanosis (severe defects present early). Hypercyanotic spells may occur due to infundibular spasm.
- Surgery is the definitive treatment: either a one-stage repair, or an initial palliative procedure (Blalock–Taussig shunt) followed by repair.
- Medical complications include high haematocrit, hyperviscosity and infective endocarditis.

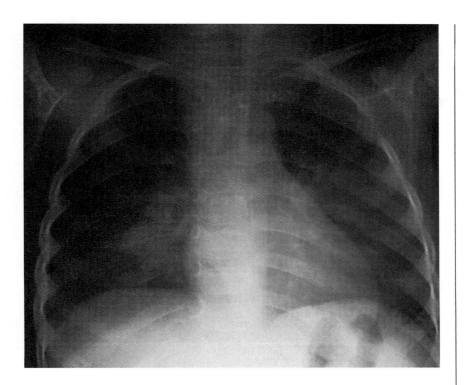

This 3 year old Bangladeshi boy was seen by his GP for persistent cough, fever and failure to thrive.

1. What does his chest X-ray show?
2. What is the most likely diagnosis?
3. What are risk factors for this condition?

ANSWERS

1. The right hilum is enlarged due to adenopathy and perihilar consolidation. There is a right paratracheal soft tissue mass displacing the trachea to the left, which represents paratracheal lymphadenopathy.
2. Primary pulmonary tuberculosis.
3. Malnutrition, immigrant population from endemic area, social deprivation and the immunocompromised patient.

RADIOLOGY HOT LIST

- Focal consolidation (in any zone) is typically associated with hilar/paratracheal lymphadenopathy (primary complex). The pattern of disease in childhood differs from the adult presentation (typically apical location without adenopathy).
- Lobar collapse may occur due to bronchial compression by mediastinal lymph nodes or secondary to endobronchial TB. Pleural effusion is present in 10%.
- The parenchymal lesion usually heals and calcifies within 12 months. However, haematogenous dissemination can cause miliary TB (fine nodular shadowing throughout the lungs).
- The X-ray appearances may continue to deteriorate while the child is receiving appropriate treatment.
- Always suspect TB if mediastinal lymphadenopathy is present in an at-risk patient.

CLINICAL HOT LIST

- The primary infection is usually respiratory due to the inhalation of *Mycobacterium tuberculosis*. Primary infection is usually asymptomatic but systemic symptoms may be present in 10%.
- Potential outcomes of primary infection:

Development of immunity	containment of infection by delayed hypersensitivity reaction and subsequent granuloma formation
Progressive primary TB	inadequate immune response with local progression of disease
Miliary TB	massive haematogenous dissemination
Post primary TB	endogenous reactivation or exogenous reinfection

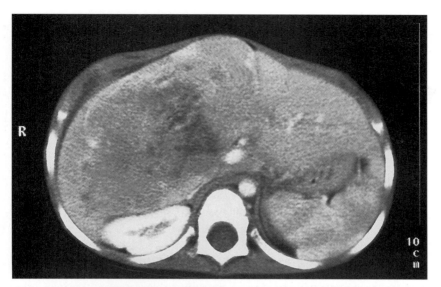

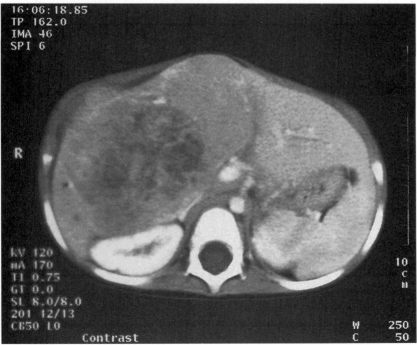

This 18 month-old girl presented to paediatric outpatients with a 2 month history of anorexia and weight loss. On examination there was a large mass in the right upper quadrant. Her serum alphafetoprotein was raised.

1. What abnormality is seen on the contrast-enhanced CT scan of the abdomen?
2. What is the most likely diagnosis?

ANSWERS

1. There is a large, ill-defined and mixed-attenuation mass within the right lobe of the liver. The left lobe is normal. The mass is displacing the surrounding organs but does not appear to invade them. The right anterior abdominal wall is distorted by the mass. The kidneys, retroperitoneal structures and spleen appear normal.
2. Hepatoblastoma.

RADIOLOGY HOT LIST

- Both hepatoblastoma and hepatocellular carcinoma appear as ill-defined, low-attenuation masses and demonstrate inhomogenous contrast enhancement. Biopsy is required for differentiation.
- CT and MRI localise precisely the position of the tumour and assess its resectability.
- The differential diagnosis includes liver metastases, most commonly from neuroblastoma, Wilms' tumour, lymphoma and leukaemia.

CLINICAL HOT LIST

- Hepatic tumours represent 1% of childhood tumours (60% malignant, 40% benign haemangioma/hamartoma).

	Hepatoblastoma	Hepatocellular carcinoma
Age	Under 5 years	5–15 years
Associations	Beckwith–Wiedemann, Wilms'	Hepatitis B and C, biliary atresia, α-1 antitrypsin deficiency, other causes of cirrhosis
Presentation	Abdominal mass; systemic features less common	Features of cirrhosis, splenomegaly, clubbing and pain; systemic manifestations more prominent
Management	Surgical excision, adjuvant chemotherapy	Chemotherapy and radiotherapy; less amenable to surgery

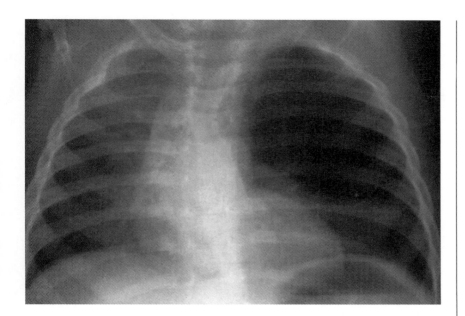

Following an uneventful pregnancy and labour, a term baby is noted to have a respiratory rate of 100 on his routine postnatal examination.

1. What does the chest radiograph show?
2. What is the diagnosis?

ANSWERS

1. There is a difference in transradiancy between the two sides of the chest, with increased lucency in the left upper and mid zones. The pulmonary vessels are attenuated in this area. There is minor mediastinal shift to the right, and the left lower lobe appears partially collapsed.
2. Congenital lobar emphysema of the left upper lobe.

RADIOLOGY HOT LIST

- Overdistension of a lobe leads to hyperlucency of the affected lobe with collapse of adjacent lobes. Mediastinal shift may occur.
- Distribution of involvement: left upper lobe (40%), right middle lobe (30%), right upper lobe (20%).
- Initially, lung fluid may be trapped in the affected lobe due to impaired bronchial clearance, producing an opaque mass on the CXR. The classic radiographic findings occur as the fluid is replaced by air.
- CT scanning can confirm the diagnosis, and exclude the presence of an extrinsic mass (such as a bronchogenic cyst) causing obstructive emphysema.

CLINICAL HOT LIST

- Localised bronchomalacia or compression of a specific bronchus leads to overexpansion of that lobe secondary to air trapping. Additionally this compromises ventilation of the surrounding normal lung.
- 15% of cases are associated with congenital heart disease.
- 50% of cases present with neonatal respiratory distress, but delayed presentation in infancy with mild intermittent symptoms (respiratory and feeding difficulties) is well recognised.
- Surgical excision of the affected lobe is reserved for those who fail conservative management.

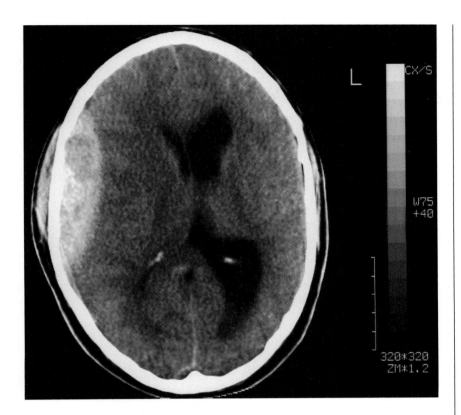

This 16 year old boy was brought to A&E following an assault. He was hit on the head with a snooker cue at his brother's 18th birthday party at the local pub.

On arrival in A&E, he had signs of a left hemiparesis and soft tissue swelling over the right frontal region. He was intubated and ventilated prior to a CT scan.

1. What does the unenhanced scan show?
2. What is the diagnosis?

ANSWERS

1. There is a large, convex high attenuation area seen in the right frontal region. This is causing mass effect with midline shift, effacement of the right lateral ventricle and dilatation of the left lateral ventricle. There is associated right-sided extracranial soft tissue swelling.
2. A right extradural haematoma.

RADIOLOGY HOT LIST

- CT is the modality of choice for the detection of acute intracranial haemorrhage.
- An extradural haematoma is a collection of blood between the dura and the skull vault, usually associated with blunt trauma to the skull.
- The convex lenticular nature of the lesion is diagnostic of an extradural collection.
- There is an associated skull fracture in 40% of cases (up to 80% in adults).
- Additional findings may include extracranial soft tissue swelling, intracranial free air (suggesting a compound fracture), and intracerebral haemorrhage/contusions.

CLINICAL HOT LIST

- All children with an extradural collection warrant urgent neurosurgical referral.

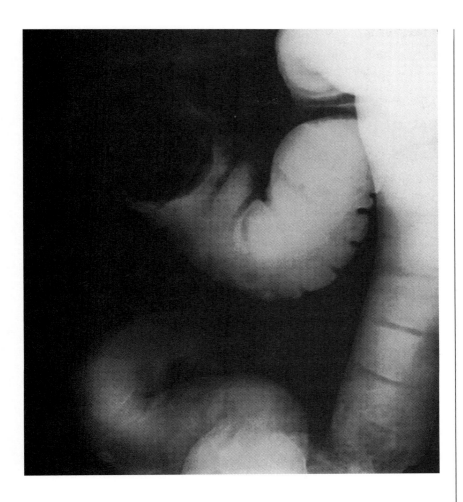

This 1 year old boy presented with a sudden onset of screaming and vomiting.

1. What investigation has been performed?
2. What is the diagnosis?

ANSWERS

1. A contrast enema. Contrast is seen in the large bowel outlining a soft tissue mass in the proximal transverse colon.
2. Intussusception.

RADIOLOGY HOT LIST

- The value of the plain X-ray is debatable. It may be normal (25%), show a soft tissue mass (50%), and/or small bowel obstruction (25%). It may be useful in excluding other diagnoses.
- Ultrasound is almost always diagnostic, showing the 'doughnut' sign. Absence of blood flow suggests bowel necrosis.

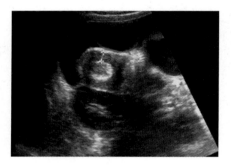

Typical ultrasound appearances of an intussusception.

- Air or contrast reduction has <1% mortality if performed within 24 hours. The overall success rate is 70–85%. Reduction becomes increasingly difficult if the intussusception has been symptomatic for more than 48 hours. The contraindications are perforation, peritonitis and hypovolaemic shock, in which case the child should proceed to immediate surgery after resuscitation.
- Recurrence occurs in 6–10%, half within 48 hours of the initial reduction.

CLINICAL HOT LIST

- Invagination or prolapse of a segment of bowel into the lumen of adjacent intestine: ileocolic (75–95%) > ileoileal (4%) > colocolic.
- It is the commonest cause of acquired bowel obstruction in childhood. It is usually idiopathic, but a lead point (Meckel's diverticulum, lymphoma, polyp, duplication cyst, Henoch–Schönlein purpura) is present in 5%.
- The peak incidence is between 4 months and 2 years (<10% of cases occur in children over 3 years old).
- Presentation is with acute onset of colicky abdominal pain, vomiting, redcurrant jelly stools and cardiovascular collapse.
- Complications include vascular compromise (bowel infarction), bowel obstruction and perforation and hypovolaemic shock.

Bibliography

Caffey's Pediatric X-ray Diagnosis. An integrated imaging approach, 9th edn. Silverman F, Kuhn J (1993) Mosby, St Louis, MO.

Forfar & Arneil's Textbook of Pediatrics, 5th edn. Campbell A, McIntosh N (1998) Churchill Livingstone, Edinburgh.

Imaging in Paediatrics – a casebook. McHugh K (1997) Oxford University Press.

Nelson's Textbook of Pediatrics, 15th edn. Behrman R, Kleigman R, Nelson W, Vaughn V (1998) WB Saunders, Philadelphia.

Non-accidental injury: review of the radiology. Rao P, Carty H, *Clinical Radiology* (1999) 54, 11–24.

Practical Pediatric Imaging, 2nd edn. Kirk D (1991) Little-Brown, Boston.

Primers of Diagnostic imaging, 2nd edn. Weissleder R, Rieumont M, Wittenberg J (1997) Mosby, St Louis, MO.

Radiology Review Manual, 4th edn. Dahnert W (1999) Williams & Wilkins, Baltimore, MA.

Synopsis of Paediatrics. Habel A (1993) Butterworth-Heinemann, Oxford.

Textbook of Neonatology. Roberton N (1997) Churchill Livingstone, Edinburgh.

Index